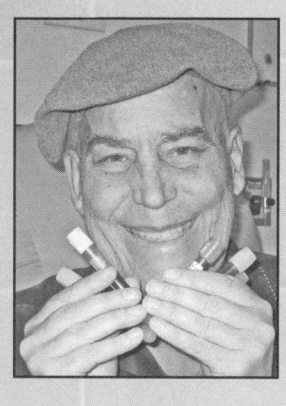
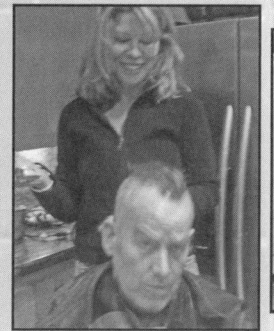
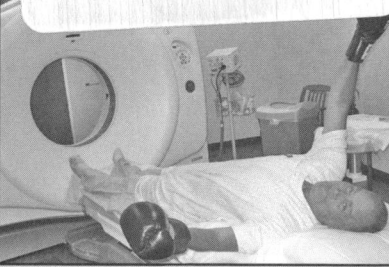
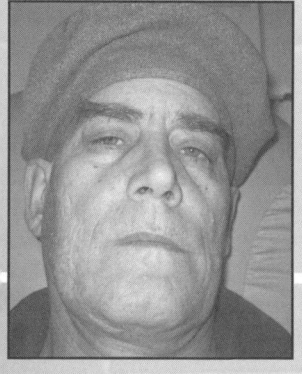
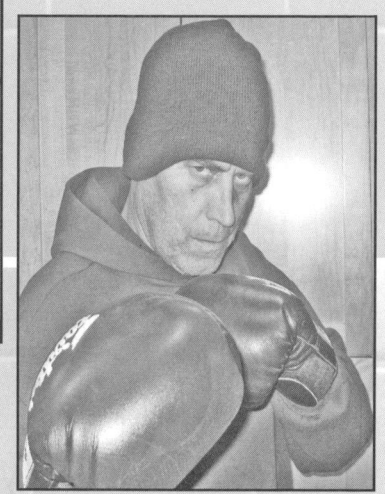
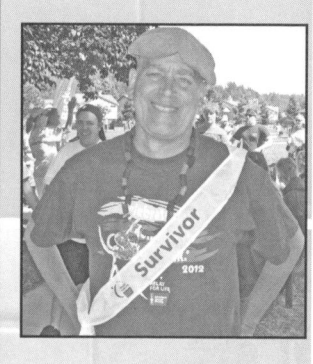
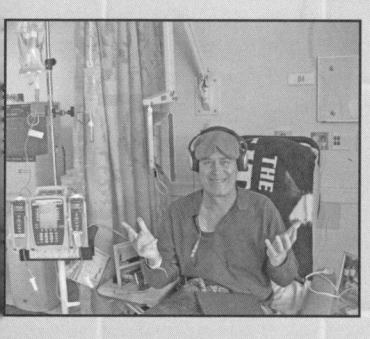
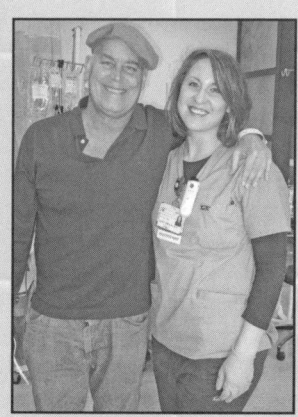
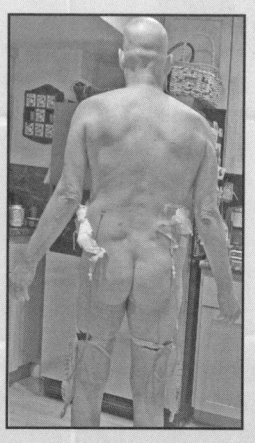

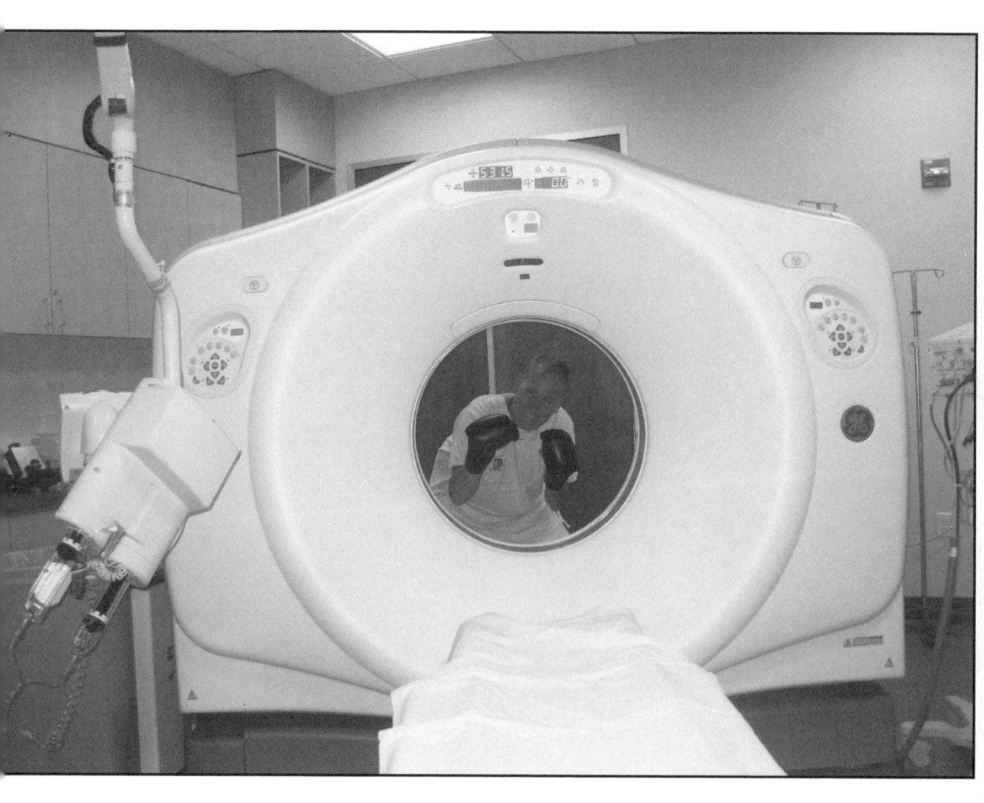

Today
Cancer
Tomorrow
The World

As *real* as *it* gets

A well-hung tale of a better life without testicles written in first-person Chemoscope.

by

Fred Reiss

Copyright © 2013 by Fred Reiss All rights reserved. Published in the United States by Santa Cruz'n Press, Santa Cruz, CA. www.fredforyourhead.com.

ISBN 978-0-9623869-5-4. Cancer — patients — United States-Biography 2. Cancer — Patients — United States — Family Relationships

Jacket Design by Frank Doyle of standingstone.com.
Type knowledge and editing kudos to Lee Yarosh and Beth Regardz.

Printed in USA.

FIRST EDITION

AUTHOR'S NOTE: This books is based on my experiences. I've changed the names of certain people. Some scenes have been condensed, but it's all true. No images of me in this book were Photoshopped. I did everything you see.

Special thanks to the tag team who cared, brought me gifts, carried my surfboard, rides to the hospital, and gave of themselves to make me possible: Laurie Roberts, Hal Stanger (who as a friend made many sacrifices for me) his wife Jody, their son Shannon, Johnny and Catherine Arbogast, Janet Herrington, Stephanie and Chuck Navigante, Ronnie Jacobson, Paul Bayon, Jack and Virginia Roddy, Dr. Zen Majuk, Mike McMahon. Wendy Mayer Lochtefeld, Marcia Rider and Gwen Marcum at the Capitola Book Cafe. Bill Farrington, Dr. David Resnick-Sannes, Mark Purdy, Lee Yarosh, Ken Dixon, Bob Moseley, John Kosowatz, Frank John Hadley, Kerry Hull, Tim Atkinson, Antonio Drexel, John Stone, Laureen Cameron, Kristen Hager, Mark Landig, Driveway Dave, Robert Berry and Rebecca Matthews-Werner, Yvette and Dave Lawson, Steve and Lynda Hall, Joey Greer (For taking out our garbage because I was too tired to do it), Terry Arnaud, Vicki Ventner (for the reflexology foot rubs!), Odwallah Ken, Brandon Armitage, Annette, David, Lena and Eva Hunt, Ron Davis, Billy Vega, John and Lorraine Schumacher, Wayne Kenney, Pat Farley, John Mel, Linda Walton (for all the DVDS), Frank Caprista, George and Pam Burgdorf, Maggie and Phil McReynolds, Greg and Jay Kihn (especially for the visits, CDs, books, mags, cookies and herbal support), Chris Jackson, Frank Doyle (For the Sorrento's Sub), Les Ginsberg (For being on call.), my brother and sisters. I hold up an encore match for Steve Siacotos (Who came to our house on Valentine's Day, took out as guitar and sang *Beyond The Sea* to Laurie and me. I was too tired from chemo to dance with her to it.). And an unending giant bow to the most beautiful women in the world: the stellar chemo-cocktail mixing oncology nurses at the Stanford Hospital's Infusion Treatment Area. And a thank you to Dominican Hospital in Santa Cruz, and the Stanford Cancer Center for my cure and forgiving the remainder of my debt left after my insurance coverage.

To a cure

&

A world of less pain without side effects

&

*Caregivers who give to others
the most valuable thing in life: their time.*

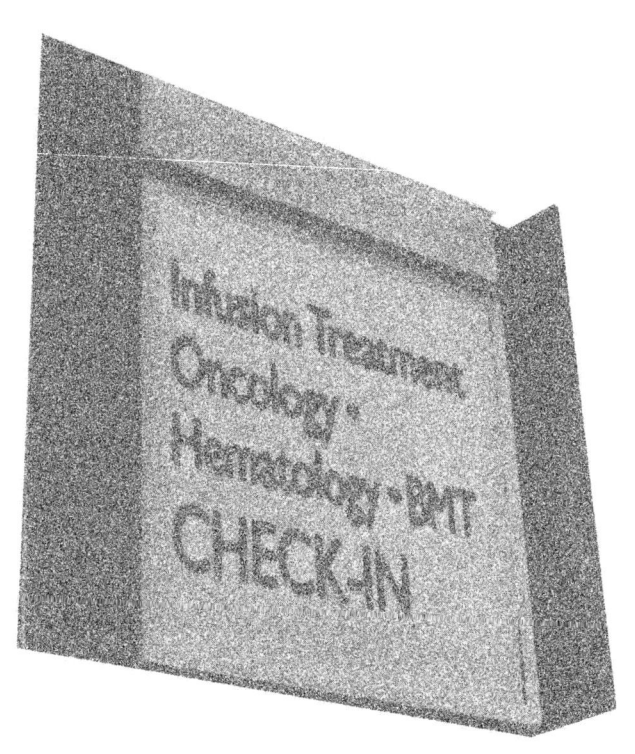

PRIMER COAT

Nobody knows where the aliens came from or how the various strains of these self-destructive beings invade the soft tissues of their future victims. They've been here since the ancient Greeks and Romans. Some believe this unknown malignant mass over the centuries is evolving mutations within the living in a quest to become immortal. This alien preys upon every living thing. It has no organs. It has no nervous system. It has no mouth — yet swallows its victims whole. It takes the lives of millions. None are safe. It devours pre-med and premees, hedge-fund managers and caregivers, soccer moms and deadbeat dads, Oscar winners and community-house players, Black Labs and Siamese cats, CEOs and janitors, Olympic runners and toll collectors, investigative journalists and public-relation hacks, mob bosses and district attorneys, junk-food addicts and health-food freaks, breasts and testicles. Once the inimical alien infiltrates its host, the creature's growth invasively expands its malignant helix-like fingerlings that latch, twist, entwine and engorge the blood supply from its victim's lungs, stomach, liver, spinal cord, pancreas, brain, colon, even tonsils — this mutant has no tongue so all organs tastes the same. Its thriving imperfect storm robustly spreads like malignant pollen and blossoms insatiable cluster bombs of clear cells throughout its prey's body, multiplying and dividing in a pincer movement, ravenously advancing and feeding at its self-catered all-you-can-eat cellular buffet. As the alien swarm robustly teems within its human habitat, their afflicted victim withers, fades away and dies. Without a life-support system to nourish the embedded alien with nutrients and a sugar rush, the mutated tumorous mass dries up, cracks open, dissolves and completes its messianic suicide mission by becoming one with its unforgiving and forever silenced host.

This repellent invader has no feelings. No family. No love or hate. No fear or remorse. No reasoning.

And it's inside me — *again*.

"**I could never go through chemo and lose my hair,**" inconspicuous people vapidly comment about themselves while I endure my cancer treatments in their presence.

You couldn't lose your hair. You really think so, huh? And you could *never* go through chemo? Or go through what I'm going through. Have catheters plugged in your back. Walk with urine bags strapped to your legs. Lose so much weight you see your skull and your belt is on its last loop and your pants are still falling off and even your feet are loose in your shoes. And you still think you could never go through what I'm going through? Well, when The Big C cold cocks you from behind, flips you over, crawls on top of you, presses one of your shoulders on the mat, and starts leaning its full weight on the other shoulder, and you're a quarter-inch away from being pinned to surrender what little you know of your life — it's then, when The Big C monstrously smiles and its foul deathknell breath is upon you — then and *only then*, will you know if you have what it takes to go through what all cancer patients go through. Some people easily go down for the count, but cancer isn't what defeats them. They respond to the malignant foe the same way they face any adversity. Without any resistance, they'd drop their last shoulder with relief if they get fired from a job, if they lose retirement in their 401k, if a spouse dumps them for another, if their home is foreclosed, whatever — and they have an endless supply of whatevers they'll surrender to without firing a single shot in anger. They easily relent, drifting into the comforting blank muggy haze of oblivion and welcome death because they believe there's a better life somewhere else. They betray themselves. Their lifesupport system is outside their heart. They were dead to begin with. During my treatment, I was told about a guy diagnosed with cancer. He had a wife and kid. He refused chemo because he didn't want to lose hair and get thin, and weak. He allowed cancer to fill in the blank. He ended up thin and bald and weak — but, without hope. I'm not him. I can't drop my other shoulder. *That's not in me.* And The Thing filling my body and trying to pin me from the inside out is going down first. Not me! I'm in no hurry to leave. Eternity can wait a while longer — a lot longer.

What is the triumphant core of light that pushes out the beam that illuminates the power of my soul and prevents the darkness from pinning me down for the count? It's not faith. It's not fear. It's the spark that lights up my smile with a sense of humor. It's what puts the special bounce in my dance step to the thumping call of a universal beat. It's what cried out of me when I was born and the doctor smacked my ass. It's the reflection that glistens when my eyes meet the eyes of someone I love. And I will *kill* for it.

Death is inevitable but that doesn't mean it's necessary.

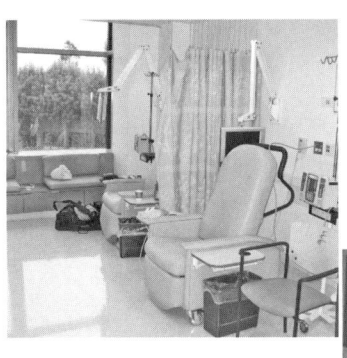
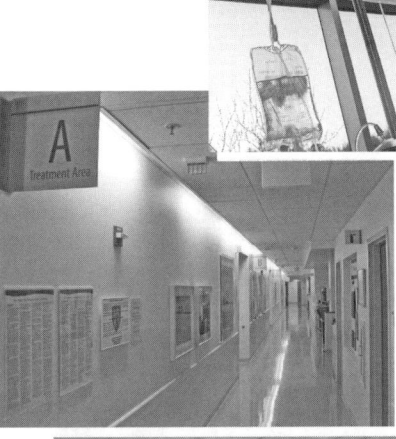
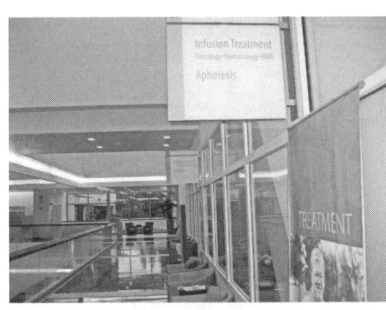
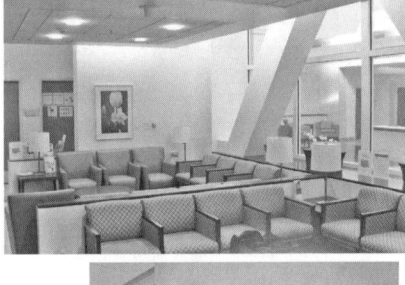
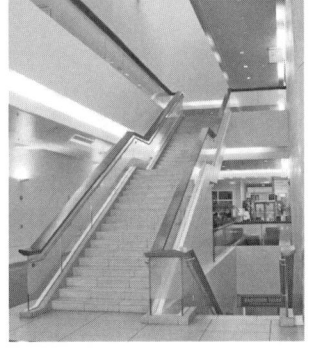
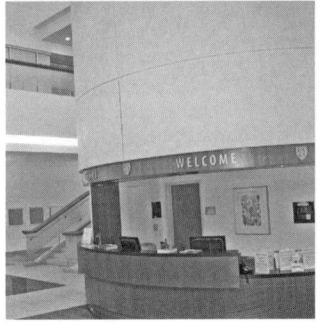

People ask me what the Stanford Cancer Center is like…

It's like the Hilton Hotel *with Chemo!*

Very good and fine chemo.

Apologies to Caregivers: no Mini Bar.

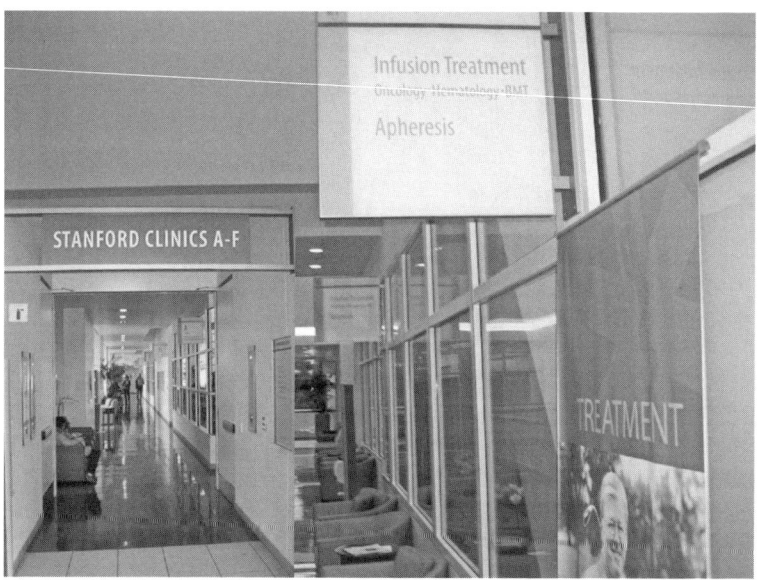

My High Noon at dawn: no one at this chemo-IV showdown except me and The Big C. What song comes into me? *Early Mornin' Rain* by Peter, Paul & Mary: "In the early mornin' rain, with a dollar in my hand, and an aching in my heart, and my pockets full of sand."

GRABBED BY THE SHORT HAIRS

THEY ARE METHODICALLY WORKING THEIR WAY TOWARDS ME. Hard footsteps followed by soft footsteps. For some reason, oncologists have hard sounding shoes and their assistants walk lightly on soft ones. A door opens and closes down the ward's hallway. I'm not the only patient they are seeing during the December holiday season. Humbled by the incoming moment. There is nowhere to take cover. I'm completely exposed on a white sheet of butcher paper attached to a roller on the examination table in one of the many rooms in Clinic E of the Stanford Cancer Center's Oncology Urology unit. My life is downsized and a tumor is outsourcing me. Cancer has turned my body into a crash pad. I'm nourishment. I'm being digested from within. My cells are fast food. I'm a happy meal. I'm waiting for my oncologist. It's our first meeting. Ten minutes later, I hear a door open and close, followed by hard footsteps and soft footsteps then another door opens and closes. I feel like I'm in a cell on death row with the warden and priest coming for me. I think of Merle Haggard's song, *Sing Me Back Home*. I want to return to the world of healthy. That's why I'm here, but not *why* I'm here.

I wait. This isn't my idea of shopping for Christmas sales. I absently flip through out-of-date news and sports magazines. Fifteen minutes later, a door opens and closes. Now, the footsteps are louder and closer. This time they enter my room.

When I look up from the magazine, I see their expressionless professional faces. My eyes begin to water. If I stare at them long enough they'll become cloud formations. I hang my head.

This is as real as it gets.

And it's not going to be good.

How does cancer happen? The same way an accident does. You turn a blind corner and in your lane there's an 18-wheeler semi-trailer truck carrying a 40-ton load. *And there you are.* Some people attempt to reconstruct their past to isolate the specific vulnerable stress point in their lives where cancer impregnated them. It's reverse conception. Where did life begin to end? They crave the illusion of an answer. Everyone hopes there is a cause so they can rationalize what created the origins of a tumor some vandalizing Darkness indifferently slapped onto their organs. *They need a reason.* They think cancer's a crossword puzzle that can be solved by going down and across. When you're sown into Cancer's World there's no longitude or latitude. The Big C doesn't need a compass to plan its vacation stay. You can't locate the malignant hot spot in your past, anymore than you can predict the joys of life ahead or business opportunities. Whatever rationalized bubble of steel the dedicated seal themselves inside for protection, cracks open when The Big C lightly brushes against it. And then you're merely another topping on life's-took-a-big shit-on-me pizza — and all you can do then is ask for thin crust and maybe a little extra cheese. Trying to understand how I landed here is like folding up a map that won't go back to its original shape. Wherever the hell I am now, I'm lost.

How did I discover my cancer? I had been vomiting after meals for no particular reason. Even when I was surfing, I didn't feel 100 percent me and missed easy waves. I was off center. My wife, Laurie, insisted I go to our local doctor. I had an uneasy feeling I didn't want to share with her. I felt the familiar inky presence of a tentacled predator inside me. I had cancer once before. And suspected a repeat performance. So, in November of 2011, I made an appointment with my GP, Dr. David Resnick-Sannes. I chose Dr. Dave because we golfed together many times. An elegant gentleman who impressed me with his politeness, kindness, self-effacing intelligence, interest in the arts, and his generosity of time caring for his patients. A dedicated quality guy. Everything you want in a doctor and a friend. He was even like this when he was golfing! Fortunately for me, he was a better diagnostician than he was at reading a green for a six-foot birdie putt. He conducted a routine exam. He pointed out the swelling in my right foot — it was something I hadn't noticed. It was significantly larger than the left. I mentioned my digestive problems. Dr. Dave took out a hand-held ultrasound device that resembled a small blow dryer. He oiled my abdomen, ran the device over it and studied a screen in front of him. He detected an "irregularity in my pelvic region" and sent me to Dominican Hospital in Santa Cruz to undergo a more comprehensive ultrasound.

I left and went to a radiology clinic. I was in a hospital gown, lying on my back, getting set for a CT scan to determine if the tumor had spread like black butter and melted throughout the rest of me. A retracting platform slid my strapped me into the holding cell of a three-foot cylinder of a machine that looked like a gigantic industrial front-loading clothes dryer. A radiologist in a sealed lead-lined control room hit a button. The machine's computer-generated voice said, "Hold your breath." Within a few minutes, the twin towers of my body and life were doing a full-on 9/11. How many people strike a pose for a photograph and know when it gets developed see if they'll live or die? I thought, is this it? Is my life over? Within this confined cylinder, I felt like I was being buried alive by my own flesh. I'm imprisoned in my own body. Tears rolled down my incarcerated face. These were the first of my many cancer tears. When you cancer cry, you don't sob and heave. Tears bead and drip out of you. They come from the back of your eyes like tap water.

Later, I realized what these tears really are: my soul is sweating.

AFTER MY ORGANS WERE MICROWAVED AND SONARED, I RETURNED TO DR. DAVID FOR THE RESULTS. When I entered the office the receptionist didn't shake me down for a co-payment. She studied my face, as if she was sketching me. Immediately, I knew from her cautiously courteous manner something was dreadfully wrong. People don't act that concerned if you're just sick.

Dr. Dave was stricken and drawn. His eyes were glazed with tears and he said in an aggrieved tone, "You have a significant tumor."

I was the calm one because he was more upset than me.

"How big is it?" I said, uneasily.

"It's about the size of a small football. I'm sorry."

"You don't have to be apologize, you caught it," I said. "If you missed it, then you should be sorry. Sometimes it goes undiscovered. You've saved my life."

"I've set up an appointment for you," he paused, then firmly added. "You're going to Stanford."

MY ORIGINAL DIAGNOSTIC OUTLOOK WAS BLEAK. The oncologists at the Stanford Cancer Center were contemplating a difficult operation to remove the large tumor, which could have adhered like Velcro to feed on the blood sources of my surrounding organs. If so, its removal required separating the healthy tissues from the tumor, and resectioning the organs. I met with an insensitive and smug urologist I'll call Dr. Guptah Rashnesh, who was appointed to do my possible surgery. He was in his mid-forties and made the mistake of thinking he was impressive as well as funny. He had the personality of a complex cheddar.

Dr. Rashnesh smirked, shrugged and cavalierly said to me, "I have done many of these operations. Sometimes the tumor pops out. Other times it attaches to organs and we resection them. We won't know what's there until we open you up. We're looking at a six-hour surgery. I might have to remove your bladder."

I spoke up, "Time! You *don't* have to remove it. You can *rebuild* a bladder."

"But that would take *another four hours*," he glibly said, shrugging.

What an asshole! He looked at me like I was a frog he once dissected in Biology class. After all, if you grew up in a borderline Third World country where it's common to find out Uncle Shankar was meditating under a banyan tree and get fang whacked by a cobra, then finished off by a Bengal tiger, I guess refusing to spend a few extra hours in surgery on my bladder and condemning me for the rest of my life to wear a colostomy bag isn't such a big deal! But my karma wasn't signing on for the all-life-is-suffering health care.

Fortunately I was given a reprieve. The callous bladder-challenged Gupta was counterbalanced by one of the Stanford Cancer Center's top surgeons. Dr. Jeffrey Norton, a seasoned man in his mid-fifties with straight-forward deep gravitas, and a considerate and focused bedside manner. He was grounded in the depth of my dismal moment. Dr. Norton looked directly at me and calmly said, "You don't want to go through this surgery. I've done them. They're very complex." I'm impressed a highly skilled surgeon was in no hurry to slice and dice me. "I want to conduct a more detailed biopsy to determine if the tumor is a sarcoma or a germ-based mass. If it's a sarcoma we'll go forward with the operation. But if it's germ-based, germ-based tumors are highly responsive to chemo. Once the tumor's shrunk, it'll be easier to remove the rest of it."

A few days later, I had a biopsy done. They poked me fourteen times.

The tumor was germ-based.

Dr. Norton did the right thing. I averted a life-threatening surgery.

That's how I found myself in Clinic E's Urology/Sarcoma unit at the Cancer Center in Palo Alto, California, looking up from an out-dated magazine at Hard Footstep and Soft Footstep.

MY FEMALE ONCOLOGIST, DR. SRI LANKA, AND HER ASSISTANT STAND BEFORE ME IN CLINIC E'S EXAMINATION ROOM. Sri Lanka is the nickname I gave her, and you'll see why I wasn't too happy with our arranged patient-to-doctor partnership. My providers, Hard Footstep and Soft Footstep looked like clay animation figures. Their neutral and benign facial expressions baked and hardened in the convection oven of past malignant conversations. Their long hair is pulled back and clenched in bun claws, as if it was tightly wound on their heads like a spring. I was half afraid the claws might snap from the strain, and sharp split-ends would whip out and blind me. Wire-rimmed glasses pressed into their faces. Their lips were straight lined — I could have hung wire hangers on them. What can I say? Their body language didn't translate into a promising moment. When Dr. Sri Lanka glanced down at my folder I had the impression she didn't know my name until she read it. Instead of making eye contact with me, she studied my file. I was one of today's many cases. I wanted to snatch my folder from her soft bejeweled hands, smack her across the face with it and shout, "Stop looking at that file, I'm right here!" But I was too devastated to resent her groove-hardened professionalism, her abrupt stop before the unlocked door of humanity. I stared dumbly at her as she thumbed through pages of flow sheets, lab results, imaging studies. Hey, what can I say? I'm not feeling the warmth.

When Dr. Sri Lanka's flat eyes finally met mine, it was like her face was painted on a billboard with a roller. There wasn't a note of concern in her detached clinical preciseness and uninflected voice over. She robotically recited my test results and medical history in a measured tone she recited many times before to others. The woman had the bedside manner of a an inert gas. She didn't see me. I'm a template reduced to a tumor. She talked to the disease. I was in her way. She asked me to take off my shirt. She percussed my back with her fingers like she was looking for a beam underneath drywall. She took a disc from the file and sat down in front of a computer on a small desk near the examination table. From what I could tell she and the computer both ran on a hard drives.

"These are the results of your second CT scan," she said.

My CT scan appears on the screen. The gray-and-white shifting and throbbing black-and-white splotches look like one of those radar pictures of an approaching storm front. Only this storm is building within my body and my cells are caught up in it, helplessly spinning like a kite snapped from its strings into gale force winds.

"There is the enlarged pelvic mass," she continued without any emotion and pointed at a big white blob amid the blackness and other grayish expanding and contracting blotches that were supposed to be my organs. All I saw was an animated Rorschach Test. "The mass has pushed your bladder to your stomach and is blocking your right ureter and enlarged this kidney. See how much larger the kidney is on the right than the one on the left? That could possibly be kidney damage. We can't determine how far it's spread because the size of the enlarged mass prevents us from seeing most of your organs."

I assumed "mass" was a euphemism for "tumor." I had been reluctantly tutored by my run through the "standard of care" clinical obstacle course and learned the underlying meaning of many words in the medical *terminal*ology dictionary. For example, "necessary medical procedure" is a euphemism for an exam that inflicts an enormous amount of pain and discomfort on a patient. "Access" means sticking a needle in your flesh. "Interventional" means they're poking inside you. I guess it sounds better then saying, "This is going to hurt because we're jabbing your organs with sharp wires and claw-clamping probes."

I leaned forward and stared at the shifting white blob on the screen. Cancer reminded me of a roommate who eats other people's food in the fridge.

"Your information shows you have had testicular cancer before," stiffly stated Dr. Sri Lanka, flipping through the pages of my file.

"Yeah, years ago I lost a testicle to cancer, so now I'm down to five," I said.

Dr. Sri Lanka blankly stares at me. Her assistant looks confused.

This is a tough room.

Years ago, that line always killed when I was Fred 28 – 40, performing stand-up comedy. Maybe these two were stunned a patient could be funny. This was my second tour of duty as an unwilling dance partner in the beatless ballroom of testicular cancer. What else was I to do? Grovel and cry?

She said, "We've had patients like you before who have had a reoccurrence of testicular cancer." Then added as if it would console me, "Some younger than you."
"What's cancer without a sequel?" I said, shrugging and smiling.
No laugh
She casually added, "After your treatment your testicle will be removed."
"There's no way around that?"
"In these cases this is what has to be done," she said.
"On the bright side, I'll never have to turn and cough again."
No laugh.
When you have cancer and can't get a laugh with semi-related dick jokes, you're in trouble. Performing on the Oncology circuit is one tough gig.

> **Testicular Cancer:** The most common cancer diagnosed in males between ages 15–34. The rate of new cases in the United States each year is 3.7 per 100,000 people. Testicular cancer has been rising in the developed countries at 2% per year since 1970. There is a variation among racial and ethnic groups, *men of Scandinavian background have higher than average rates of testicular cancer,* African-American men have a lower than average incidence. Testicular cancer occurs in three age groups: boys 10 years old or younger; males between the ages of 20 and 40; and men over 60. *Men with a history of undescended testicle have a higher-than-expected incidence* of testicular germ cell cancers. A man's lifetime chance of getting it is about 1 in 270. The risk of dying is 1 in 5,000. 80-90% of cases will recur within the first year of diagnosis. The vast majority of the remaining 10-20% of patients will recur in the second year after initial management. *Late relapses of germ cell cancers have a unique biology and clinical management. Such patients probably should be seen at a center of excellence.*

I HAVE TESTICULAR CANCER FOR THE SECOND TIME AT AGE 57. I'm typecast in a bad remake. At first I thought the odds of getting testicular cancer again were astronomically higher than 3.7 in 100,000. But in "contralateral" testicular cancer involvement, the odds are actually higher by five percent! "Contralateral" is a medical term meaning two similar organs opposite each other. Don't you feel better knowing that? I didn't. Cancer doubled down on me. Really, think of the chances of getting testicular cancer twice! I'm on a roll. Maybe, I should play the lottery today. I guess if you get testicular cancer the *third* time, you're either a carnival act, a highly in-demand porn star, or an alien. My existence has been reduced to a very unlucky statistic. Thirty years ago, when I was diagnosed with testicular cancer, I didn't fit the profile then, or now. I never smoked I'm not even have no Scandinavian blood. My Dad was German, and mom Polish. When he invaded her on their 1954 honeymoon, I was born. On top of this, I didn't have an undescended testicle. Hey, I'm a guy. My body is descended *from* a testicle!

Depending on when it's discovered and the type of tumor, testicular cancer has a high-cure rate. The odds are supposedly in my favor. But why believe statistics for a cure are on my side? When cancer has your number, there is only one number: you! You're the *one* person who has it. Odds mean nothing. The doctors asked me if there was a "history of cancer" in my family. Double duh! Who doesn't? Cancer took my Mom and Dad. But I had cancer *before* they died. Thirty years ago, I received radiation treatment for the disease. Could the fallout from that treatment caused cancer to reappear? Radiation mutates cells. Later those cells can become benign or malignant. When I drilled down and went data mining, each new factual nugget about cancer or my treatment was countered by what could go wrong and result in a permanent side effect or fatality. Years ago, doctors put leeches on people to bleed them for a cure, and I wondered if one hundred years from now, radiation and PET/CT scans and chemo will be viewed the same way. I read an article that said the medical profession still uses leeches on patients, but I bet it's to shakedown people to pay an overdue bill.

"Radiology will call with an appointment for PET," said Dr. Sri Lanka. "It's important to see if the disease has spread. If there's involvement in other places, such as the liver, I will prescribe a different chemo cocktail. We will schedule you as an outpatient at the Infusion Treatment Area versus inpatient-direct admission. The most likely chemotherapy we will give you is carboplatin-etoposide versus cisplatin-etoposide depending on creatinine function."

I asked, "What's the difference between the CT scan and the PET scan?"

"The PET scan uses glucose. Cancer cells like glucose. We need to find if cancer advanced to your liver. A liver doesn't have glucose, so if glucose shows there —"

I snap, "If it's in my liver, I might as well hang it up and walk out of here."

"No, no," said Sri Lanka. "The biopsy revealed you have a germ-based tumor, which is highly responsive to chemotherapy. Because you previously had radiation when you were first treated, this time…we have to do chemo."

"Chemo," I uttered and imagined myself hooked up to a machine, skeletal, deadened and bald, wasting away like a concentration camp prisoner.

"You have four cycles."

"Cycles? What's a cycle?"

"A cycle of chemo is five straight days in Infusion."

"How long with I be there?" I asked, figuring I'd be in a chair for an hour or so.

"Six to eight hours," she said.

"Oh, six to eight hours, five days a week?" I said haltingly, as if I expelled my response after being smacked by a steel bar in the stomach. "Will I lose my hair?"

"Yes."

I stared at my shoes and pressed my lips. I sat in one place but was free falling. Sometimes you don't need gravity to hit bottom. It comes at you sideways.

"But before you do chemo, you have hydronephrosis. Your creatinine is elevated. You will need a bilateral nephrostomy."

Not only was I told I had cancer, they were speaking to me in another language. I was stranded in a foreign land and couldn't read the street signs.
"A what and a what and a what?"

> **Hydronephrosis:** An the abnormal enlargement of a kidney. It results when the flow of urine is blocked in the ureters connected to your bladder.
>
> **Nephrostomy:** A catheter tube placed through your skin and into your kidney. The tube drains urine from your body into a collecting bag outside your body. It is performed under ultrasound guidance, CT fluoroscopy or under image intensifier. Local anesthetic infiltration is used to numb the area where the needle would pass through to make the puncture on the kidney.
>
> **Creatinine:** a compound formed when food is changed into energy through metabolism. Creatinine tests measure the waste product creatinine in blood and urine. These tests tell how well your kidneys are working.

Dr. Sri Lanka professionally downshifted into automatic pilot and spoke like she was reading a cue sheet, "Hydronephrosis because your right kidney is enlarged due to the mass blocking the ureter. Chemo is very toxic and if it doesn't flow through the kidney properly it can permanently damage the organ's tissues. Your creatinine level is extremely high at 2.4 and the normal level is 1.3. We have to get your creatinine down so your kidneys can handle the flow of chemotherapy. In their current condition they would be damaged due to the toxicity of chemo. A bilateral nephrostomy is a medical procedure that involves inserting a catheter through your back and placing stents inside both kidneys to drain the urine through tubes that will go to drainage bags outside your body."

"Like a colostomy bag?" I slowly asked, feeling like I've been reduced to muck.

"It's temporary. You'll be required to wear the bags throughout your treatment, about three to four months. We'll start sometime in January and you ideally conclude your treatment in March."

"I'll have to wear those bags that long?" I sighed, shaking my head.

"You'll wear the bags for a couple of weeks before chemo, until your creatinine levels are acceptable to handle the chemo. Then, you will be scheduled for four cycles, separated by two and a half weeks to recover from chemo."

I say nothing because she is talking to the tumor not me, so, I didn't want to interrupt their conversation. I couldn't help but resentfully think she spent maybe what, one or possibly two hours going through my data and determining my care? After what? Reading and seeing a couple videos? What is this open-mike night? I'm not auditioning for her. *She's* auditioning for me. I angrily wonder how many unnecessary future tests and duplicate scans I will also have to endure so all the additional doctors along the way can protect themselves from malpractice suits, regardless of the pain and strain they inflict on me? You know, it's like the way people step on a spider, pick it up with tissue paper, crush it again, and flush it down the toilet — stepping on the bug once was enough to kill it, but crush and drown it too? The only difference between that spider and me is I'm alive *after* I get stepped on, crushed, and flushed with chemo.

When I thought of all the medical procedures ahead of me, I imagined Dad at my side, his hand on my shoulder and whispering, "Fritzie, don't let them do to you, what they did to me."

Dad's cautious words are a deeply implanted conviction within me — a core of resistance and presence. He will be with me throughout this. When doctors are trusted, we saw the damage they could do — and walk away from, unharmed, stuffing our money in their pockets.

"You might want to look into banking your sperm," added Dr. Sri Lanka.

I was tempted to ask if she took direct deposits. But didn't go there. I wasn't going to bank. I didn't have kids and never wanted any. Talk about finality, huh? My sperm and I had achieved closure.

"Do you have any questions?"

I decided it would be better to visit the Infusion Treatment area before I had to go there. It was a way to cushion the toxic shock.

"Where is Infusion?" I asked.

"It's upstairs."

"So, can I see what it's like before I *have* to go there?"

"Certainly, if a nurse is free she can give you a tour. We will schedule an appointment next week for your nephrostomy," she quickly looked at her watch. "If you have any further questions you can contact my office."

Dr. Sri Lanka and her assistant briskly clumped out with their folders. Departing hard flat heels followed by soft steps went up the hallway. The next door opens and closes. Their monotone voices rattle off uninflected procedures and malignant demographics to the next poor sap on the Clinic E Disassembly Line. I'm left on the examination table. I feel like her accurate diagnosis has trapped me in a room filling up with black water. It rises over my head. I limply sink, anchored to my body and impassively watch my air bubbles wobble to the surface and pop. I'm swimming in Death's touch tank. Anger and fear can't alter my situation — my emotions don't have that luxury, they must go somewhere else, have to. But where to?

My tumor weighs in at four pounds.

I didn't want a cancer encore. But I couldn't deny it. I was washed ashore on a naked atoll where if I lied to myself, I wouldn't survive.

I'VE BEEN VAPORIZED INTO A MINE FIELD OF CELLULAR DEBRIS. I'm no longer me. I've been pounded out like a piece of veal and slid into a folder:

> **Clinical History:** 57-year old male with history of left testicular cancer in 1981, status post left orchiectomy and radiation to the pelvis. He was found to have a pelvic tumor displacing the bladder with bilateral hydronephrosis. The measures 13.2 cm. in AP dimension, 11 cm. in width, and 12.6 cm. in craniocaudal dimension (3; 272 and 602; 69). Mass extends beneath the bifurcation of the abdominal aorta into the lower pelvis along the right pelvic wall. The mass causes proximal bilateral hydroureter. Significant mass-effect on the adjacent bladder. Moderate bilateral hydronephrosis is present. Some mass-effect on the adjacent bowel and colon without evidence of bowel obstruction. The mass encases the right iliac artery and vein. Biopsy and pathology showed likely germ cell tumor. Scrotal US demonstrated in the right testicle a homogeneously hypoechoic, well-circumscribed lesion measuring 1.1 x 2 x 0.8 cm. concerning for a germ cell tumor. Demonstrated large FDG avid pelvic mass, retroperitoneal lymphadenopathy, and hypermetabolic left supra-clavicular fossa mass compatible with metastasis.

What is this wow-and-fluttered haunted world of daylight gleaming off the hospital's tiled floors and towering white walls? I'm skidding in a deadpan from my ruins in Clinic E. I'm diminished. I'm like a piece of live bait on a hook in a strong current, bouncing on the bottom. *Drifting along with the tumbling tumbleweeds.* I turn down into a hallway of enfeebled, stricken, patients, stooped unmanned vessels. *See them tumbling down.* Careening distressed calls. *Pledging their love to the ground!* Every other person looks like they're staggering away from an explosion. *Lonely, but free, I'll be found.* I'm discharged and pass clinic waiting areas with letters on signs at their entrances. *Nowhere to go. But I'll find, just where the trail will wind. Drifting along with the tumbling tumbleweeds.* I'm going in a reverse alphabetical-clinical scale — E, D, C, B, A, while those on the way to be diagnosed — A, B, C, D, E, F. Turn off the shopping-mall like hallway. The letters reveal their true identities: Breast/Clinic Surgical Oncology, Urology/Oncology/Sarcoma, Radiation/Neuro-Oncology, Lymphoma/Hematology/Gyn Oncology, Head & Neck/ Gastrointestinal oncology, Brain Tumor. *Drifting along with the tumbling tumbleweeds.*

In the waiting lounges are anxious, aggrieved patients laid off from their lives, innocent in spirit but forced to appear at a clinical trial where negative results mean you're fine and positive results mean you're sick. Then why do they tell us to think positive? Oddly, the patients' caregivers look even *worse*. They're overweight, out of breath, limping, pale and coughing. And they're supposed to be healthy ones!

There are small lounges across each clinic's waiting area. In the lounges I sometimes saw a masseuse, or a musician softly playing a guitar. But today, what do I see? A glum woman plucking a harp. Yikes! Harps are not reassuring after I've been diagnosed with a malignant tumor. At least the harpist isn't wearing wings, a flowing robe and ascending to the ceiling as she weaves her hands in a circular motion across the harp's strings. She looks like most classical music majors Fred-20 knew at Antioch College. They're morose, thin with straight hair and wire glasses or pear-contoured with radish-shaped heads and oily hair draped over their skulls like an stiff paintbrush. A harp in a cancer center, hello? I guess she replaced the guy who wore the skeleton costume, black robe, and gave directions by pointing his scythe at the chemo area — he probably got promoted by corporate to run the Human Resources department. A harp! Are they trying to tell me something? A harp! Why? If the oncologist has bad news, do they say to an assistant, "Cue the harpist when I tell the patient, 'You should get your affairs in order and walk towards the light.'" And who the hell listens to a harp unless they don't have a pulse? A harp is the last instrument I want to hear. I need a reason to live not be uncomfortably numbed into gazing at my boarding pass to the everlasting kingdom of an Elysian Field's gated community in the sky. Count off! One, two, three, four! Lay down a pounding backbeat, bring in a wailing sax, hot-ripping-feedback-squealing guitar solos, heart-thumping bass runs and a screaming down-on-his knees R&B soul-drenched singer! A death-defying sound to put dancing in the limbs of my legs arched with the muscles of a howling wolf screaming for the yipping dawn of endless tomorrows. Make me furiously alive in this sick antiseptic wilderness of bright lights closing the darkness around me. Free me! Who the hell surrenders to a celestial sound check? When it comes to harps, I'll sit out that cherubic chord change!

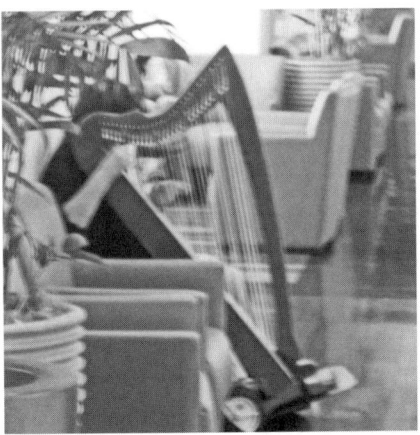

A harp is the last instrument a cancer patient wants to hear.
Why don't you just tell me to walk towards the light, flap my arms and end it?

There are thirteen days left for Christmas shopping, but no holiday decorations adorn the Stanford Hospital's Cancer Center's door There's no mistletoe either. I balefully stared at the stark sign:

> Infusion Treatment Area
> Oncology Hematology BMT
> APHERESIS

Nice wording! I guess they don't want to discourage walk-in traffic with:

> Chemo Area
> Cancer & Blood Filtering
> Leukemia Bone Marrow Transplant

That's not exactly warm and fuzzy. No matter how you spell it or say it, the signage will never have as much curb appeal as:

> Steak
> Seafood
> Cocktails Dancing Nightly

"Oncology" instead of *cancer*. "Infusion" instead of *chemotherapy*. "Hematology" instead of *blood*. "BMT Apheresis" instead of *Bone Marrow Transplant*. The phrasing might be medically euphemized, hot waxed and sanitized but it didn't change my circumstance. I felt chastened for an offense I didn't commit. I've been taken into custody. Deported into the subdued world of displaced humility. Cancer doesn't plea bargain. In a few weeks, if I want to remain alive, I must go through these doors. I uttered the first of many groans blended into a moan and a gasp, a different note of "mmm." It's the sound when something takes a bite out of your life. I'd expel it many times over the next several months.

"This is a fuckin' miserable day," I mutter, hang my head and place my hand on the warm door handle.

I enter the Infusion waiting area. Its décor is pretty upscale on the stress-free side. A lot of dangerous dark wood. A reception desk gives the impression you're checking into a four-star hotel. Yeah, the Hilton *with chemo*. A flat screen on the wall flashes images of harmonious nature — beautiful landscapes, dolphins. Artificial plants are by windows that view the outside hallways. Soothing pan-flute music plays on the speakers. You'd almost believe it was a lounge for a spa or a crematorium. It's a combination of both. People put their life on mute and *have* to be here or die. The room's ambience is subdued and unsettling. It feels hermetically sealed from the interior, not the exterior. Everyone looks depleted in this pressurized cabin. Vacuum packed by nothingness. Slam dunked by circumstance and shanghaied. They are waiting to be called for their chemo-party-of-one seating reservation. Soon I'll be sitting among them for a scheduled departure and arrival that ends up in the same destination. The room's atmosphere seemed like it hunkered everyone down in the chill of a low-lying fog. It's easy to tell the glumpy Chemosabis apart from caregiving family members or friends. Yeah, Chemosabis, I got the term from 'Kemo Sabe,' a nickname Tonto the Indian, gave The Lone Ranger. The Chemosabis wore knit caps pulled down on their foreheads, showed no expressions. They are staring to a place within their lives that's beyond this room. A few are bone marrow or leukemia patients with weakened immune systems who must wear cloth face masks with vents on them, which gives the impression they're downed pilots — in a way, they were. Most were sullenly slumped in their chairs, worn-down by treatments. They are dull-eyed, disheveled and look like they tumbled out fully dressed from a dryer in rumpled and frayed baggy shirts, and shabby sweatpants popping with lint pilling. The caregiving civilians on the healthy side of life were traveling tourist class: absorbed in laptops, reading newspapers or magazines, checking cell phones for messages, doing crossword puzzles, yawning or drinking coffee. No one was speaking.

    I walked up to one of the mahogany-framed walled booths. A smiling woman sitting behind a black-marble counter. She could have been a courteous bank teller. I looked down at the floor, then at her and said, "I'm scheduled for chemotherapy in a couple weeks, and I wanted to be given a tour, if I could."

    "I'll see if a nurse is free to give you one," gently replied the woman.

    A few minutes later, an oncology nurse introduced herself. I trailed after her. She opened a nearby door to the treatment areas. We walked through three co-ed communal infusion rooms. Large windows overlook trees but the views are obstructed by construction equipment making improvements to the hospital. Each room had about eight stations with reclining chairs and small flat-screen TVs on swivel arms. Every station occupied by a patient radiated a respectful and softened edged circle of seared isolation, like each person was a lone survivor in a chair thrown free from an airline crash site. I didn't want to disturb anyone. I somberly walked outside the Chemosabis' perimeters, trying to avoid eye contact with anyone, fearing they might glance at me with distrustful or angry eyes. I didn't want them to think I was sightseeing. I saw a wide age-range of weary, powerless and resigned people connected to tubes from clear chemo sacks hung on poles as clicking and humming computerized monitors slowly pumped a continuous infusion into their veins. The process looked like their bodies were being drained not filled. I noticed a man in his late sixties, gray hair, crumpled in a recliner, his eyes slits, mouth turned down. Like he was dissolving. His distressed wife beside him, a grave, taut-strained tension of suffering deeply carved on her face, and a copy of *Forbes* magazine in her lap. In another recliner, a drowsy middle-aged Mexican woman had a knit cap on her head, its woolen topped knob looked like the nipple of a baby's bottle. Her lower arms streaked with purple bruises from needles. Others drearily stared at nothing as nurses held bags of chemo and read the patient's bracelet and stated their name and birth date while another nurse entered the data on a computer. One nurse said, "I'm switching out the Mannitol." I heard another say she had to "hang some chemo." I was surprised other Chemosabis looked fine. I thought everybody would be whacked out. Quite a few patients were hooked up to chemo like they were being refueled. They were reading books, watching TV, listening to iPods on headsets, using laptops or iPads, chatting to visitors or playing games on their cell phones. I followed my infusion docent down a hallway past a private rooms with beds. I spot a middle-aged woman. She wasn't sleeping. She was conked out. A brown wig askew on her bald head. A resolve began to wind, knot, and harden in me. I thought, no matter how tired and beaten chemo makes me, *I'll never lay down for cancer* — never. The Big C won't catch me sleeping at my post.

"Well that's it," said the nurse after our three-minute tour, smiling.

Back in the waiting room I passed quietly slouched, wrung-out Chemosabis. They were distant but immersed in their surroundings. Dark planets orbiting the Sun of Hope. Ironed-out dismayed refugees in an alien country. We were more like self-exiled pilgrims in an uncertain frontier. I'd soon be one of them. My reality has taken off on another flight. I was booking passage to Another World.

AFTER VISITING INFUSION, I'M SUCTIONED OUT OF THE HOSPITAL LIKE A POPPED-OPEN BLUR. The trees in the mild breeze made an angry pneumatic hiss. Gnarled dried leaves slowly scratched the concrete sidewalk. On this pleasantly warm and sunny California day, completely engaged medical staff and students ride bikes, jog, sit on benches and eat cafeteria food from Styrofoam trays in the courtyard. Some dressed in scrubs, others in white lab coats, jackets and ties, walking rapidly, talking on cell phones and laughing. I'm close-up but appraise them from my new outpost. Preoccupied people doing what they're doing and involved with whatever they say in a temporary time. When you're ill, the world drifts about like a floating joke. I feel everyone is deluding themselves they're not circling my eventual landing area. Any open display of health mocks me, unless it acknowledges my suffering. Every activity is a value-added fraud. I'm not part of their transitory extracurricular-outdoor activities. My life is split by a fault line into two regions: healthy and sick. I'm roped off from the health section and segregated among the sick. The healthy stand and dance in front of me, blocking my view of the show. Have they ever traveled to distant worlds without taking a step? Feared a collapsed pulse? What is the voice that makes these puppet on the strings take this stage? And so I wonder. Caught in the grasp of the helpless. Carrying the chemo cross. I have no time for equal time. I watch them and I was once one of them. If I break free from The Big C and come back to the halo of another life, I know I won't be the same. Somehow I'll drift alongside them in a different current. I guess lateral promotions do work. I hope it'll be an improvement — or at least have a better scenic view, even though it's probably all done with mirrors. I'll never be one of these people again. Returning here will be like adding another 88 keys on a piano and wondering what tunes I'll play that I never heard until my hands touch the keys. A second chance to never be who I was. "Doc, if I survive cancer will I play ever be able to play the piano again?" I ask. "Yes, I don't see why not?," replies the doctor. "Funny," I say, "I never did before." Bada-bing!

EVERYONE DESERVES A SECOND ACT TO CHANGE THEIR LIFE. I call it the Scrooge-wakes-up-on-Christmas-and-buys-the-Cratchits-a-goose moment. Some experience an emotional catharsis going through their first firefight, a serious illness, or the traumatic loss of a loved one. Some get belated epiphanies on their deathbed. Fred-27 was lucky to be given a second act. Unfortunately, most people are deprived of a second chance. Dad didn't get one. Mom didn't either. And another patient whose name I can't recall was denied his appeal too. But I owed him big time. Years ago, when I was getting radiation for testicular cancer, I was in a room awaiting treatment. A bald, skeletal teenager with a brain tumor sat across from me, resting his head on his distraught mother's shoulder. His cancer was more *advanced* — odd use of the word: advanced. He held an expensive camera she purchased for him — you know when you're going to die because people go out of their way to give you the gifts you've *always* wanted. I told him I was a newspaper reporter. He said wanted to be a photographer.

He asked, "So what kind of cancer do you have?"

I replied, "Testicular."

He smiled, his hollowed eyes hardened and he weakly said to his mother, "Mine's different, huh?"

She started crying.

He looked at me with a glare of accusation. I knew what that creasing penetrating stare meant: "When you leave here, what are you doing with the life I'm not going to have? *You better do something with yours.*" After I finished my last radiation treatment, his presence trailed me — he was the foreman on a ghostly jury of haunting peers who didn't make it. Sometimes when I kicked out of a wave or told a joke on stage that got a laugh or said something funny on the radio or finished writing a book or simply came home to Laurie, I imagined his thin figure, intently studying me, nodding. Thirty years later, here's Fred-57, out of work, and diagnosed with cancer again. But the plot-twisted life I created came to rescue me. I lived near Scotts Valley, 45 miles from the Stanford Cancer Center in Palo Alto. Laurie couldn't take me because she started a new morning radio job at KPIG, a cool Americana station in Watsonville. I needed rides to-and-from the hospital for chemo throughout four separate five-day week periods spaced out through January and March, as well as additional rides to go for tests during my two-and-a-half week furlough period between chemo tours. Laurie and our friend Lynda Hall teamed up and put together a sign-up sheet on the web. In ten minutes my friends filled slots and volunteered for one-hour rides — that reaching out brought tears to me, and can still do it. No one even asked for gas money. Cancer can be a blessing. That's hard to believe. It's like being alive and getting a privileged chance to attend your funeral and discover if you lived right. And I *have*. My friends rose up in arms to defend my life. Their overwhelming support and love and concern and calls and emails and gifts and cards from others endowed me with an additional reserve of strength. My somewhat estranged sister Cynthia even sent me five hundred dollars. With all this support rallying behind me, I knew when I stepped into chemo for the first time, I was running on far more than my own power. I wasn't alone. My feet were propelled by the tailwind of a million-man march.

TODAY I'M MODELING THE LATEST IN BUTT-CRACK HOSPITAL GOWN LINGERIE FOR MEN on the fashion runway of another examination table. I don't think butt cleavage is a plus. Today, my kidneys are getting fitted for a nephrostomy. A middle-aged Irish nurse ignores me as she checks my vitals, then winds a rubber cord on my right arm like she's wrapping a package, and routinely sticks a needle in me as she gabs with another nurse about where to go on their lunch break. Amazing. Oddly, her detachment amuses more than offends me.

I said to the nurse, "I have to get these tubes. The tumor is blocking my ureters. I was diagnosed at the Cancer Center last week."

She testily snapped, "You know, there are *other* things being done at this hospital, we are more than just cancer."

"I'll keep that in mind," I said, surprised the distinction meant more to her than my plight.

The nurse started my IV, drew the curtains and went off with her coworker to lunch. On the gurney, I'm introduced to one of those unavoidable intermissions between the hospital process and life. My clothes and valuables are stuffed in a paper bag. The only thing to identify me is a hospital bracelet. Sometimes in our lives there's a loaded silencer pointing at us. We're in the lapse between our pulse or phone calls or books or today and tomorrow. I'm pinioned by The Fates in a gurney and waiting for either the doctor or an attendant to take me to the procedure. All I can do is wait and think. I'm left with dry and empty stretches of prolonged seconds and straining minutes where I can't read, watch a movie on an iPad, or go online or listen to music on headphones. I'm floating, suspended in a balloon of nothingness. There's a lack of continuation when cancer puts your body on a deadline. It's like facing the present blindfolded.

I shake off the nippy unwelcomed snuggle of the present, and say to myself, "Where is this taking me?"

Everyone goes to a different place in their lives during these coerced intermissions. When Fred-27 had cancer, I laid in the hospital gurney with an IV-needle in the soft blue vein of my right arm. I thought, if I get a second act, who will this guy be when he's lying in a gurney again? It was life altering. Fred-27 pledged to go to California, do stand-up comedy, surf, and go to Australia. I never made Australia, but three out of four's not bad. After I finished radiation and saved enough money, I quit my job as a reporter at the *Danbury News-Times* in Connecticut and never looked back. The perks and trappings of a newspaper career meant nothing to me. I set out to live the life of my heroes. Like Kerouac I drove cross-country to California. Like the cool California lifeguard Tommy Chambers I worshipped as a kid, I learned to surf. Like all the comedians I admired, Mort Sahl, Lenny Bruce, and Don Rickles, I performed as a stand-up comic all over the country and on national TV. Like Jean Shepherd and Don Imus, I became a humorous radio talk show host and interviewer. Like Thoreau, Steinbeck, Hemingway, I published a few books, and one novel won a PEN award, another was optioned by actor Nicholas Cage (And like most things out of Los Angeles, nothing came out of it.). *But I still built a life!* It was important to me, because Dad was a corporate guy and relocated with his company a few times. In retirement, he envied men in town who ran a local business and remained in one place because they had known each other since high school and formed deep friendships. Outside of golf partners at his club, Dad didn't have any real buddies. If Fred-38 wanted to continue his stand-up career, I'd have to move to L.A. and lose the roots I established in Northern California — my surf and golf buddies, the woman I loved, and everyone else along the way. I decided to walk off the stage to pursue a radio career and writing. But when Barack Obama got elected in 2008, Clear Channel radio suits used the victory as a smoke screen to bury in the news their announcement the company was laying off 10 percent of their long-time employees. It might have been 10 percent to them, and since I wasn't one of the suits compiling the list, 100 percent of me went out the door. All the bad guys kept their jobs. Laurie, a successful rock DJ in the South Bay for twenty-five years, also lost her gig. I did fill-in radio slots and found a part-time job as a tasting room manager at a Santa Cruz mountain winery, which turned out to be incredibly rewarding. I wound up working a crush, making my own wine, and creating an even wider circle of offbeat but passionate friends. In between scavenging for a paycheck and collecting unemployment, I wrote novels and figured I was due for a break. A cancer rerun wasn't exactly what I envisioned as my next career move.

Here was Fred-57, with testicular cancer again, an IV-needle in my right arm, lying in the exhausted fumes of my fulfilled dreams. Throughout my life, what was I really the best at? *Being me!* Who isn't? Well, now I had a chance to prove it — again. After getting a taste of my left testicle, cancer is going down on me for my right one. Now I know how Captain Hook felt in *Peter Pan*, when he heard Tick Tock the crocodile. Tick Tock ate Hook's hand and liked the taste and wanted to eat the rest of him, but the crocodile also swallowed an alarm clock. Its ticking warned Hook of the crocodile's approach. The ticking I hear is different. Is cancer trying to run out the clock on my meter? I need a crocodile game delay.

I flash to an old memory. Fred-24 in a suit on a train station platform, commuting to NYC from Westport, CT to a copy writing job at Macy's. I was terrible at it. I feared writing sales copy would contaminate my ability to be a real writer. I resisted producing anything of quality. I only took the job because my girlfriend was living in The City. After I was hired, she broke up with me. While I waited for my ride, a Norwalk train from the opposite direction, dropped off black women who came to clean the Westport homes of the commuting businessmen, whose wives were shopping or going to the theater later. My legs straddled a crack in the concrete platform that marked where the train stopped and where its automatic doors slid open. Other guys in suits were clustered in their chosen spots for different doors. Soon I would see the approaching train banking around the bend, reflecting a flickering sliver of sunlight on its windows. Almost everyone had a newspaper, but I carried novels. I didn't know what I really wanted out of life yet, but if I read novels those words remained with me forever, and might form a solution, while reading the newspaper would get me through the day, but never show me how to tunnel out.

And now I lie in a gurney, atop my cracked world looking for any train of thought to take me anywhere but here. I try to shrug off the twitching pain of an embedded IV spidering its splinter legs in my arm. It grates on me. I'm agitated.

I buried my face in the crook of an elbow and sheepishly bleated, "Oh shit."

WHO'S NEXT? I'm transported on a gurney in the hallway to the operating room. I'm pushed by a guy named AJ. I'm lying there like a baby in a crib, looking up at the passing ceiling lights. AJ weaves through medical staff, who are on cell phones, most of them see us, but don't move out of the way.

I said to him, "Boy, she didn't do a thing to make that turn easier for you."

AJ grunted, "Happens all the time. Doctors are the worst. Some stand in the middle of the hallway and don't move. They think they're so important."

I said, "A friend of mine is a respiratory therapist, he told me the more important the organ the bigger the asshole."

"That's true," said AJ, nodding.

I said, "Before a doctor gets hired, they should have an IV stuck in their arm and wheeled in a gurney from one end of the hospital to the other. And then spend one whole day in a clinic with that needle in their arm."

"That's a good idea."

"I can see doctors saying it's undignified if they had to do that. No more than me or anyone, who never wanted to have cancer and be in a gurney. Maybe doctors have to see the world they look down upon to understand why some people don't look up to them."

"You're sure a talker, aren't ya?"

I'M FERRIED ON A GURNEY TROLLEY INTO THE OPERATING AREA LIKE A BUFFET SERVED UP BY ROOM SERVICE. The staff is upbeat and friendly. One nurse cheerfully greets me with, "Welcome to our office!" They *revive* me. I'm reactivated. I start goofing on the procedure and we're all laughing. They put a blood pressure wrap on my arm to monitor me and I said to the nurse, "I'm like you, this is not the first time we've been squeezed by an inanimate object." They crack up. Another nurse says she wears an iPod while she vacuums her house. I said, "So you don't hear the rats in your place?" A guy says, "She actually *does* have a rat in her apartment." Then I added, "Which ex-husband is that?" They all laugh. She says, "I'm just unlucky in love." And I quip, "With your personality I'm not surprised." They say, "We want this guy back!...Too bad we have to put him under, we want him to keep talking." I ask, "Am I being put under?" "No, you'll just be between being asleep and waking." I replied, "I always wanted to know what it was like to be a Republican."

I'm lying sideways. The drugs hit. My mind shaft is stuck between the floors of here nor there. The doctor is sitting to my right, intently staring at a fluoroscopic guidance screen to "advance" a .018 Nitrex wire into my kidneys. During the stint installation I feel a jab. My body jerks.

"Did you feel that?" asks the doctor.

"Let's just say I know you're there," I said, feeling the drugs levitate me into shifting prisms and smears of half-heard conversations.

AFTER THE PROCEDURE, I'M EASY BAKED WITH MEDS. The nursing staff caters to me. They offer me apple juice with ice. It's like being spoiled when you're a kid with a cold and you love the attention. I thought back to Fred-9. I had the mumps. Mom and I left the doctor's office and passed a drug store display window that included two plastic toy ships, a black freighter, and the USS Hope, a pure white ship that saved people. I stared at the boats. They were $1.99. I wanted the USS Hope for my bathtub fleet. Mom noticed my interest. Later that day, I was in bed with a fever. Dad entered the room with a boat, but it was the black freighter. I wailed, "I wanted the USS Hope!" Dad left and returned with the USS Hope. When I started to get better, I didn't want to lose the attention. After all, I wasn't going to school, and outside of having to go to the bathroom and missing out on TV, I wanted to prolong the drug of being healed. When people feel sorry for you it's a great high, I think that's why losers lean towards self-pity to entrap people into conversations. And you know what? After I got over the mumps and put that USS Hope boat in the bathtub, it capsized! But what did I get out of that plastic ship? A prolonged and deep admiration for how Dad indulged my childish selfishness. I imagined Dad standing at the foot of my hospital bed, a worried look on his face, holding out a boat of hope.

I kept waking up every other hour in my hospital room. The tubes filtered out my kidneys. Pain pills pulled up my moorings. Thoughts and images flashed and disappeared before I can register them, like the way sunlight fleetingly gleams off fish in the water before they disappear in the depths. Parts of me are rising up. It's reverse sedimentation. And emotions and feelings from the past and views I currently hold, float or sink. My brain is being pressed in the blood of my heart so my thoughts have *feel*. I sort through various emotions and the ones that continue and acknowledge a life that moves forward are light and float, and the ones that deal with unfinished arguments, anger, disappointments, rejections and hurts, become gray and heavy, sink and disappear — it takes an effort, a pointless mission to salvage them for they contain no riches, just bitter passengers who decided to go down with the ship.

I drifted in and out of sleep. I put on my headphones and played Todd Snider's music on my iPod. The song lyric that lingered came from *Greencastle Blues*:

> *Some of this trouble just finds me.*
> *Most of this trouble I earned.*
> *How do you know when it's too late?*
> *How do you know when it's too late to learn?*

The next morning, I was connected to something outside of myself. Twined in tubes. The catheters in my kidneys felt like I had toothaches in my back. I delicately turned in bed to avoid snagging the tubes plugged into me so I wouldn't yank out a connection. The looping tubes attached to my body make me feel like a kite that couldn't catch a breeze, then spun, crashed and was lying in the mud, tangled in its strings. I mournfully studied the urine trickling into the clear drainage bags strapped to my legs. I murmured my mmm-groan-moan-gasp. I'm a science project. The IV spidering on its splintered legs, twitched and dug into my flesh. It tormented me. When I was a kid, how many times did I visit uncles dying of cancer in the hospital? They had IVs in their arms. Dad had one. He died. Mom had one. She died. *Now I had one too.*

A nurse enter. She was in her thirties, attractive, had long black hair. She was everything Dr. Sri Lanka was not, caring, attentive, and funny.

"I'm from India."

"You didn't have to come from that far, I could have got someone who lived closer." I asked. "Can you hand me my cell phone?"

"The hospital charges $10 a minute to use cell phones."

"What?" I said, stunned and offended. "It's a cell phone, how could —"

"I'm joking," she said, giggling. "Nobody gets it. I think it's funny."

I burst out laughing. I took life too seriously and missed the joke. *That's funny!*

"How are we doing?"

"When can *we* take this IV out?" I said. "They depress me."

"The doctor has to write a release order before I can remove it."

"I hate this IV," I said, raising my arm. "I can handle going through chemo but having an IV in my arm for eight hours, five days in a row. I *know* I can't hack it."

"Your oncologist didn't tell you about a medical port?"
"She didn't offer it."
"Well, it's an option if you don't like needles."
"Outside of my heroin addiction I really have no use for them."

She smiled, then lowered her voice as if we were conspiring together and said, "I'm a cancer survivor and a health professional. For six months my doctor — not one here — said nothing was wrong with me. I went to another doctor. He found cancer. Our doctors are bright, but never forget they work *for* you. They have to do what you say — and they *hate* that. You have to be your own advocate."

"I hear you," I said, puckering my lips and frowning.

I was incensed. My oncologist never even considered a port could alleviate my discomfort. How much time does it take any oncologist to simply say, "You're going to get a lot of needles for blood and scans and have an IV in your arm for prolonged periods. You should consider a medical port." How much time would that take? Two minutes? I had to *advocate for one*? I can't cure myself, but I can *minimize* my pain.

ARE ONCOLOGISTS' BRAINS BENIGN FROM HANDLING MALIGNANCIES? Does that cause their hearts to divide and mutate like cancer cells so they eventually don't feel the pain a patient experiences? Oncologists have a lot more in common with cancer cells than they'd care to admit. You'd be surprised how systemic their professional disease is. They've studied so diligently, sacrificed, and confused maturity with arrogant pride and delude themselves that the achievement of *becoming* a doctor is sufficient enough so their personality never extends beyond themselves (Except perhaps, their stock portfolio, or accelerating their downswing on the first tee.). This self-made inhibitor justifies their abruptness to patients because these oncologists mistakenly believe maintaining an emotional distance enables them to determine the most effective treatment for cancer. They're proud of it! It's a flaw they've turned into a badge of honor called "pull-yourself-up-by-your-bootstraps." This immune system protects them from being infected by caring for a patient. Oncologists are like functional alcoholics: they don't believe they're the problem, everybody else is. Never mind how the patient actually *feels*. People who have never been *really* sick defend an oncologist's emotional shortcomings by saying, "Maybe they're overworked and haven't seen their families. After all, doctors deal with so many people. They see cancer every day. If oncologists took their work home with them, they'd have a mental breakdown." *But I've never heard a cancer patient say that*. Yes, these doctors see cancer patient after cancer patient every day. And why? Because they're oncologists! Why should a patient expect the oncologist to become emotionally involved? Well, let's see…because *they're our oncologist and we might be dying!* But these same clipped professionals don't mind forming an emotional bond with our money. Money they earn from our blood and treasure, as well as the pain and suffering that accompanied our cure or worse. I doubt if a doctor ever says, "Because my patient trusted me and they died, that failure is a reflection on my professional ability to be more effective and trustworthy to future patients. I'm refunding their money so the deceased's family won't lose their house." If doctors drop their professional distance when they spends my money, they can *afford* to spend the time to care for me. Maybe it would be better if there was a two-year gap or so before they went to med school so they might develop some grasp of humanity beyond the fluids and ingredients listed on their medical degree's box. There's no substitute for compassion. It's more than part of the healing process — *it is healing*. If I died, I'd like to know my oncologist cried. I hope it ruins their day. It showed they *cared* about me. Yet oncologists justify developing detachment as a professional coping mechanism from the horrors of cancer, but they're neglecting one key point: cancer patients don't have the *same* luxury. Oncologists don't have to take their work home, but *we go home with their work*. We can't take a day off from cancer and play golf on Wednesday. We can't put cancer on hold when they don't return our calls. We can't easily go to sleep at night, if they fail to promptly give us test results because they weren't "in clinic" the day when we were *at* the clinic. And when they get a three-day weekend or a National Holiday off, we can't stop metastasizing.

I simply say to them: You chose to be a doctor. I didn't choose to have cancer. I *outrank* you.

ANY PORT IN A CHEMO STORM — A MEDICAL PORT. When I was diagnosed with cancer, the word went forth, and friends put me in touch with others who have gone through chemo. And people who had cancer gave me guidance and advice. So many post-chemo veterans told me if they were educated about medical ports *before* they underwent treatment, they would have chosen a port instead of being jabbed with a needle every day. Many showed me how shot the veins in their arms were after chemo. Others described the pain of a nurse not being able to "stick" a vein. Another said her mother was getting chemo, and a nurse thought she had found a vein, then walked away. She didn't. The chemo burned the flesh off her mother's arm. It wasn't too comforting for me to learn the hospital didn't dispose of empty chemo bags, special Hazardous Waste Materials crews trucked it away. That was enough for me to avoid needles.

I made an appointment for a medical port. I went to the Interventional Radiology clinic on the Cancer Center's third floor. I met Ryan Daugherty, an acute nurse practitioner, a hippie-looking guy somewhere in his forties, who clearly had a sensitivity attuned to one-on-one caring. Unlike the doctors, he didn't maintain a zone defense, he believed in man-to-man coverage. He had a kind focus. He held up a display model of a half-inch port that had a plastic tube.

"Did your oncologist tell you about a port?" he asked.

"No, I found out about ports from others and decided to get one for myself."

Don Body Armor to Take Out Cancer

- Hate IVS in your arm?

- Fear Needles?

- Can't stand Blood Transfusions?

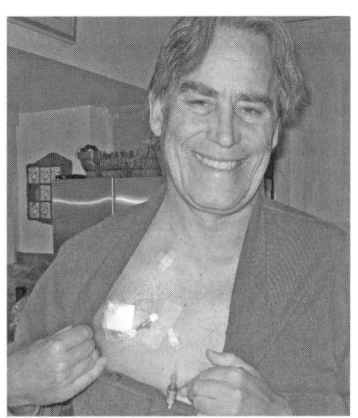

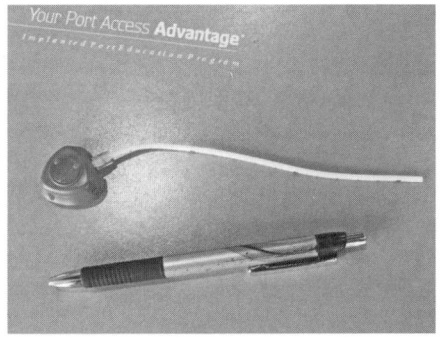

Reduce your *Pain* and *Stress*.
GET A MEDICAL PORT.

When you fight cancer
To **THROW** your best punch
Your arms *must* be **FREE!**

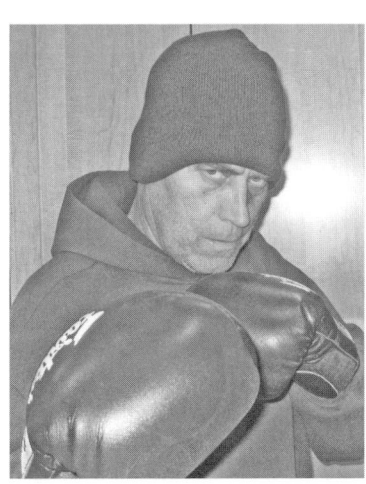

"You did this yourself," Ryan said, impressed. "Good for you. Most people don't know about them. They should."

> **Medical Port:** A port is a small medical appliance that is installed beneath the skin. A catheter connects the port to a vein. Under the skin, the port has a septum through which drugs can be injected and blood samples can be drawn many times, usually with less discomfort for the patient than a more typical "needle stick." The device is surgically inserted under the skin in the upper chest or in the arm and appears as a bump under the skin. It requires no maintenance and is completely internal so swimming and bathing are not a problem. Patient is sedated but awake during surgery that lasts 1 – 2 hours. Once implanted, the port is accessed by a Huber needle.
>
> **Huber Needle:** A specially designed hollow needle for implanted ports. A Huber needle has a long, beveled tip that can go through your skin as well as the silicone septum of your port's reservoir, causing very little damage or injury. Before chemo, patient numbs their skin with a lidocaine gel. A nurse painlessly snaps needle into place. Needle is attached to a six-inch clear tube with a connecter on the other end where nurse can attach chemo, test tubes for blood draws, hydration bags, or dye for scans. (*See Page 28.* Huber needle is taped to my chest. It's removed at the end of each week.)

Ryan spent a lot of time explaining every aspect of the device. The port is my chemo-extension cord with a plug. He considerately asked what activities I did, then said he'd positioned the port slightly above right collar bone so I could still surf or play golf with it in me. The surgery took almost two hours. I was awake during it. He slipped the port under my flesh and connected the tube to a major vein — veins are like elastic pieces of licorice, once the tube pokes into it, the vein seals around it. An hour before a nurse "accesses" my port for chemo, Ryan said, I should apply lidocaine, a numbing gel to the surface, because it takes awhile for the gel to work. The slight bump formed by the port under my skin looked like a growth. I was happy to have it in me. I was relieved to reduce one major stress point. No more needles and IVs in my flesh. I felt great.

If I was going to throw my best punch to fight cancer, *I must have my arms free!*

FOR THE NEXT COUPLE WEEKS, PEOPLE WERE CURIOUS ABOUT MY NEPHROSTOMY TUBES. But when I lifted up my shirt, they were grossed out by catheters taped to my lower back. They turned their heads away like I was a disfigured victim and sharply blurted, "I don't want to see it."

I was offended by their repulsion, but restrained myself and explained, "You're looking at these tubes and urine bags from the outside in. I'm looking at them from the inside out. I don't see the bags as gross. The bags are my knapsack I need to reach the summit. The tubes are ropes I need to climb out the well of darkness to the light." Others inquired about chemotherapy, then when I started to explain it, they'd get squeamish, shuddered in revulsion, and interrupted my answer by saying, "I don't want to know!"

I accepted the way they were. That wasn't the real problem — the real issue is *they* accepted who they were.

AN HOUR AFTER I HAD BLOOD DRAWN AT THE CANCER CENTER, I had an appointment with Dr. Sri Lanka to see if the blood tests results showed my creatinine levels were low enough for me to begin chemo. I went to the cafeteria to get a muffin. When I went there, I remembered getting a lunch when Dad was in the Norwalk Hospital, slowly dying from an infection he received from a botched operation. I had been going to see him so often, I knew the hospital's daily menu specials. It's depressing inside knowledge because it means something is wrong, like if you know all the car mechanic's names at a repair shop. Dad died because our family trusted his attending physician (Now, there's an oxymoron.) The surgeon expressed a confidence in his abilities but concocted a different explanation to cover what "little wrinkle" happened after each unsuccessful operation to correct his mistake. This was the result of trusting a doctor our family originally didn't feel right about, but bowed to his professional expertise. It's similar to meeting someone who wants to be your friend, but you just *don't feel it inside you.* There's an underlying distrust and lack of confidence that prevents the bond from being genuine. And usually, your instincts are right. I was bugged by Dr. Sir Lanka never calling me at home after my nephrostomy, and for failing to inform me about a port.

Dad's voice was with me, "Fritzie, don't let them do to you what they did to me."

"I know Dad, I know," I whispered. I decided to do something about it.

After a nurse took my vitals in Clinic E's examination room, I heard the clip-and-clop approach of hard and soft shoes in the hallway. Dr. Sri Lanka greeted me, looked at my file and said my creatinine levels dropped to an acceptable level for my kidneys to handle chemotherapy, which would begin next week.

"This is good news," she said.

"My only problem is I don't know what color shoes match my urine bags."

No laugh.

They stare at me. Tough room. It reminded me of a comedy gig I had in a British Columbia dive bar performing to a rowdy audience of anti-Semitic, Asian-hating lumberjacks and Alaskan King Crab fishermen who were on crack or meth, some couldn't flip me off because they were missing middle fingers.

"I would like to get another oncologist," I said.

Dr. Sri Lanka bristled, surprised by my directness. She curtly rattled off, "Well if you don't want to continue with me as your attending physician we have to reschedule an appointment with another oncologist, and start the whole process again. And that doctor may proscribe a different cocktail."

"You're going to give me chemo anyway, so what's the difference?"

"It'll only be a week delay. It won't really matter," Dr. Sri Lanka huffed.

She didn't know I was standing beside my Dad. We weren't budging. It felt good to be angry. No matter how nice you are, you have to bark once in awhile to let people know you're not on a leash.

"No!" I said. "I don't want to wait a week. I want to fight this cancer now."

"That's the process," she said, as if the matter was settled.

I leaned forward and said very slowly with a malevolent flat low trajectory, "Don't *I* have a say in this?"

There is a silence. I'm hoping I filled the room with a menacing afterglow.

Dr. Sri Lanka backed down and grudgingly complied, "Yes, you do."

"Then I take chemo next week. *That is what I want to do.* I'm taking responsibility for it. I can do that. I don't question your treatment. This thing is growing inside me and I want to stop it and go after it now. I don't want to win arguments. People make mistakes. I accept that. The main thing is that we all work together for me to get the best care to heal. That's our goal."

"Fine," she said, miffed.

I suspected Dr. Sri Lanka's indignation was because my request reflected badly on her track record. But I wondered if I wasn't her first dissatisfied patient.

After she left on her low heels, I imagined Dad, supportively patting me on my shoulder, and saying, "Good going, Fritzie."

Dad died in his early eighties after four colon operations and 100 days in the Intensive Care Unit. He couldn't speak. He had a trac. When they changed his dressing, I could see his insides. His unhealed abdominal area looked like a grizzly bear clawed him open and skated on him with razor blades. The one-foot long over six-inches wide gouge in him was probably larger than that, but the wound was held in place within him by plastic arched girders. The scarlet gooey gorge was stuffed with gauze. When they redressed Dad, he softly groaned in pain. I knew the gash was never going to close and he was going to die. Strange as it may sound, I was also disturbed by whiskers under his nose. I never saw those hairs before. Dad took pride in his appearance, and was always clean-shaven. His loss of dignity was because of someone else's failure. His body was hospital waste that was still too warm to be tossed in the scrap heap.

"Your father will die in a few days," effortlessly said the Norwalk Hospital ICU head, a guy in his late fifties who was bald, had wooden eyes and a pasty face that looked like it was sloppily smeared with a tongue depressor on his skull. He had the beside manner of funeral director at an airline disaster.

I said, "Did you see what you did to our father in there? We brought you a car in for repair, and you smashed it into a tree."

"There was nothing improper done, these things happen," the ICU head said.

"So, if you didn't do anything wrong, then why don't you go in there, look our father in the eyes and tell him that because of what *you did* he's going to die?"

"The most important thing is closure, and to make your father's last days pleasant," he said in an empty voice that sounded like it came out from a tube.

I wanted to punch him. I think he was hoping I would. Then he could dismiss me as irrational. But I wasn't the one in denial here. Instead, I calmly thought, *I'm going to fuck you so deep, you'll never know what hit you.*

After the ICU director left, I saw Dad. He trusted me — then I lied. As an adult, I never lied to Dad. The doctors wanted me to lie because they wouldn't admit their mistakes. I gave Dad the impression nothing was wrong. To convince him, I claimed I came back again from California to Connecticut to help with his rehabilitation. Over the next couple of days, my sisters, brother and I watched him fade as a rising stain of an infection clouded his body. He died a different shade of color every second. Dad believed he was going to make it until the day before his last. His flat eyes became reflective. He looked at me, lifted his arm and fluttered his hand. I knew what the gesture meant. Years ago, when Dad visited one of his golf buddies in the hospital, he asked him how he felt, his friend lifted up his arm and fluttered his hand: it was the sign of angel's wings flying away. Sometimes at night, or early in the morning, when I wake up, I think of Dad in a hospital bed, unable to leave. I still see his flat eyes from morphine, his fluttering hand, and I cry. I wasn't going to let the surgeon get away with what he did to our father. *They made me lie to Dad for something they did.* My siblings and I retained an attorney and initiated a malpractice suit. The surgeon wasn't there when Dad died, but he made sure he was *there* for the autopsy. In a deposition, he stated he "didn't remember being there." They want me to attain closure? Taking a piece of their reputations and money for their incompetence and killing Dad, there's *my* closure. And they can choke on it every day they look in their half-empty bank accounts for the rest of their lives!

It's important to be a good patient. I listen with respect to doctors, but I'm too guarded and skeptical to ever completely trust them again — they're made of flesh and bone too, and sometimes flesh and bone lies. Dad follows me on every hospital visit. He stands behind me, hands in his pockets. My guardian angel is packing heat.

In the empty room, I get up from the examination table. Tears form. My voice cracks into a whisper, "Yeah, Dad. You and me." I whimper. "You and me."

THE DAY BEFORE MY CHEMO BODY SOAK, I PARKED MY CAR ON 38TH AVENUE AT PLEASURE POINT. For well over twenty-five years this was my surf spot in Santa Cruz, California. I walked across East Cliff Drive and sat on a bench along the bluff's edge. I removed my shirt but covered the tubes in my back because I didn't want to upset people passing by me. I looked at my break. A guy in a wetsuit sprinted from the beach, jumped on a longboard and prone paddled into the ocean, completely stoked to surf. How many times had I been that guy? Will I ever be him again?

Ever since I was a kid, I *belonged* to the surf. Fred-12 purchased the *Surfer Girl* album by The Beach Boys because a guy named Tommy Chambers was a lifeguard at the Stonehurst Swim Club and Cabana in our housing development in Freehold, New Jersey. Tommy was from California and while he was on duty at the pool he constantly played the album on the club's speaker system. He was so cool! He scuba dived and had a spear gun. He had blonde hair and blue eyes and surfed. He showed us pictures of naked girls sent to him by real girls! Our pictures of naked women were centerfolds in *Playboy* magazines we kept hidden in our rooms between our mattress and box spring of our beds. But these were *real* women he *actually knew* who wrote sexual notes to him on the photos. And I thought what's it really like out there in California? I went home and stared at myself in the mirror. I was tan, had blonde hair, and blue eyes too. I thought I don't belong in New Jersey. I should be surfing in California. I believed, if I filled this missing piece in me it'll would link me to other places. This was the seed of my beginning.

I came to my ocean for strength. They say the sun is bad for you, but it's always been energizing for me. Time for soul broasting. When Fred-14 came home from mat surfing at Manasquan, I'd stand in the shower, kick off my swimsuit and watch the sand swirl from my body over the white webbing inside my trunks and down the drain. The water from the shower stung my sunburned flesh. I've always left the beach toasted, lighter, bluer-eyed, blonder and stronger. The sun offers light not criticism. I always felt healthier here. I needed to take this with me into the hospital. I looked at my surf spot. Tears striped my face. All those rides and wipeouts and my surf buddies who coated me with a protective dream into a more determined person and reinforced my passion to write and become a funnier stand-up comedian and endowed me with a sharpened and keener perspective angle on life to stand up for what was rightly mine — it was out there. So many laughs and barbecues and surf trips and hooting for each other's rides and standing up for one another in the water against rude morons. Surfing fed my soul. I stayed close to it. I believed the surfing life will save me. It was more than a belief. *It was a faith.* I leaned back on the bench and surrendered my unarmed body to the sun, never giving into the shade to pursue my even tan of survival. That's why I'm sitting here now. This place made me cool. I wanted to stay cool.

"Fred, you need any plants?" shouted Driveway Dave, snapping me out of my sun daze. He got the nickname because years ago, after his divorce, he lived in a van parked in a nearby driveway. He was a good-natured guy. Now, he was in his late sixties, retired from driving a truck and stacking merchandise on shelves. He spent his days hanging at the beach, throwing a ball for Blake, a dog he adopted or who adopted him. Dave always offered anyone candy, bottle water, his beach towel — even his board. Dave talked to anyone who moved — or was trapped — within his radius. They were rarely short conversations.

I turned. He stood by his van, waving me over. He opened the van's back doors. There were all these different plants and some flowers. I spotted a dried and stunted stub of a nearly dying cactus in a Popeye Spinach can. Its distressed touched me. When Fred-6 watched Popeye cartoons, I asked Mom to buy spinach. She did. I took one bite and hated it! Still do — and I especially distrust people who like creamed Spinach, they're duplicitous. I vividly remember anytime Popeye was nearly defeated by Bluto, Popeye squeezed a can of spinach and a leafy stream shot up in the air into his mouth and gave him super-human strength. The can made me get the plant. I have cancer and the cactus isn't too healthy either so I figured we spend our time growing together.

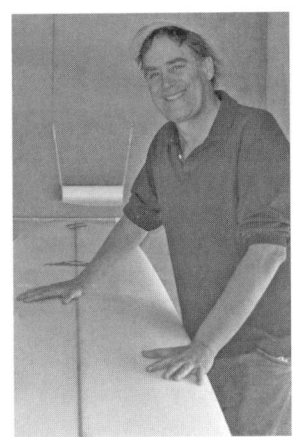

I was out of work, broke and faced with chemo and cancer. I was at the lowest point in my life. There was only one thing left to do: *buy a new surfboard!* Before you go to chemo, purchase something for your passion's future use.

———————

AFTER I LEFT THE BEACH, I NEEDED ANOTHER GOAL BESIDES NURTURING A PLANT. I used money from my eBay sales and purchased a new surfboard. It was more than a board. It was my destination. When I got home, I placed the unridden stick on racks in a back-yard shack. I ran my hand along its smooth rails. My eyes teared up and my lips quivered. With amen fragments between my fingers, I softly uttered an mmm-groan-moan gasp, and said to The Great Unknown, "I will come back — *please.*"

Sometimes a journey doesn't need a compass.

ON MY WAY HOME, I RENTED THE DVD OF ROCKY TO WATCH ONE CRUCIAL SCENE. The scene I *needed* to see. Early in the first round of Rocky's fight with Apollo Creed, Rocky unexpectedly throws an uppercut and drops the cocky champion. It was a punch Apollo didn't think Rocky had. It was the punch that meant this was a *real fight*. I needed to be able to find that uppercut in me. My life had to become a fist. I watched the scene over and over and imagined delivering an uppercut to cancer, standing over it, waving my boxing gloves, watching its writhing slime sprawled on the mat, crawling, stunned, unable to get up. I watched that fight scene over and over and over again. Now, I had to become that punch every second in every minute of every day.

My cancer tears came like sweat. I'm giving my soul a workout. I'm in training for the fight of my life.

I'm slumped at loose ends from tubes. I'm sulking in a chair by the kitchen table. Laurie is making a pre-chemo dinner to cheer me up. A barbecued rib-eye steak with a baked potato. We've been together for close to twenty-five years — she'd probably give me the exact amount of years, days, hours, and seconds. Tonight the supper mood is altered by a melancholy mildew. Henry David Thoreau had it wrong, sometimes "the mass" makes men "lead lives of quiet desperation." My hands are in my lap. My legs feel the warmth of urine flowing down tubes and filling drainage bags. I'm heavily grounded and withdrawn, wearing another layer of flesh, blankly staring ahead, mentally contracted, wondering what's going to hit me. I'm tumbling backwards in a sequel of suspended growth and watching an accident happen in slow motion.

"What's the matter?" she asked.

"I've had cancer before. I know what's ahead of me. I'm in a gurney at the top of a roller coaster and looking down at the track that leads to the entrance of a haunted house filled with scalpels, blood, and needles."

"That's not being positive."

"But that's what it *is*."

"You can't think that way," she said, her voice faltering.

"But, you have to see what *this* is. I mean, I plan on making it out. But there's no way around it. You've got to see cancer for what it *is* so you can fight it."

"You fight it by being positive."

"Fine," I said, slamming my fist on the table. "Okay, fine! You're right. You win. Let's stop talking about it."

I see my curt answer hurts Laurie. *But be positive?* My battle against cancer has *nothing* to do with positive. Because, if I concede there's a positive, I have to allow for the *existence* of a negative. I have no place for negatives. I'm not a battery in the neutral corner of pluses and minuses. There's nothing positive about fighting for your life. My pulse is a charge. It doesn't take sides. The thrumming instinct to survive is recklessly beyond positive and negative. It's something else entirely. I'm on patrol like a grunt soldier walking point in a thick jungle. I'm not positive or negative. I'm just trying to stay in a zone to remain alive. You ever see those nature shows where a calm lion has its shifting jaws clamped on a squirming zebra? The poor zebra is still alive! The lion's eyes have no affect, flat, not reflective. No soul. Just a killer. That lion is Cancer. I'm the zebra. I'll tell you one thing, when I work my way out of this lion's mouth, I'm coming back one mean-ass, cold-blooded, lion-eating zebra! And I'll tear that lion apart, rip out its bones, and then I'll piss on it. You call that positive? It's not. There's nothing positive about it — it defies positive. And I guarantee that when you find yourself washed ashore in the dark unknown of familiar surroundings, stranded on that unwelcoming pale plain of a No Man's Land on Chemo Island, and see that lion coming at you, positive is the last thing you will ever be.

Laurie suggested, "You should go to a group of people experiencing what you're experiencing. They have workshops to help people."

"I know what I'm going through," I snap. "I really don't need anyone to tell me how to feel."

Again, my answer hurts her. I wasn't proud of it. She doesn't hear me because she isn't in my world. But I was incapable of agreeing with her. So I say nothing. Cancer has locked me down in a defensive mode. I dug into a deep space in my body. Nothing was going to draw me out. I had to become my own human shield. The hardest part of explaining what cancer is doing to you is when you describe it, you become the disease and feel like you're giving cancer to someone else. I'd rather keep it inside me than spread around that particular joy.

I'm having post-traumatic stress while I'm experiencing what's going to give me post-traumatic stress. I've had cancer once. And what kind of an edge does it give me? Nothing. Thanks for nothing.

THERE WERE FALSE FRIENDS AND ACQUAINTANCES WITH VAGUE OFFERS OF UNFULFILLED SUPPORT IN MY BATTLE AGAINST CANCER. I slapped away their going-through-the-motion backing track of empty sentiments. We all have these people in our lives. They believe they're nice people — they *have* to.

"You're in our prayers," was their most familiar refrain. "We'll pray for you."

I've heard *that* phrase before. Sometimes I thought what they really meant was they were praying for themselves. *We'll pray for you.* It almost sounds like a veiled threat — you know, we'll prey for you, we'll prey upon you. I heard that phrase many times the first time I had testicular cancer. Fred-27 was lying on a slab of a CT scan machine to determine if the tumor spread to other organs.

A middle-aged nurse with a huge gold crucifix displayed on a necklace outside her uniform said, " I'll pray for you, the Good Lord will get you out of this."

I replied, "Well, He got me *here*."

She bugged me. People who experience a severe tragedy like the loss of a child might need faith to get through inconsolable grief. Regardless of what religion someone has, if they need it to get through life, fine. I mean, who am I? But, from where I sat, life was too chaotic and unfair to ignore the unpredictable and unsolved algebraic and geographic horrors inflicted upon the innocent by distancing myself with a theorem of faith that exempts me from healing the unbearable pain within the suffering of others. But oh, how those uninvolved people will *pray* for you! And how you'll be in their prayers. *Like it absolves them from doing nothing* beyond making a phone call or inquiring about your health. Hell, they'll pray for me to live. And if I die. They'll pray to the Lord for the courage to maintain their faith. It's a win-win for them and a lose-lose for me. I've never been big on religion. I don't want to draw on my 401K in the afterlife. I'll spend it here. Even if they're atheists. How do *they* know more — or less? No matter what religion a person has, they always have some out-there view of eternity. What can I say when some clearly disenfranchised but fervid born-again zealot engages me in a conversation and says, "The two preconditions have been met for Judgment Day. Israel is restored and Jerusalem is Jewish. All that remains is the rebuilding of the Third Temple and seven years of tribulation, followed by the battle of Armageddon when St. Michael will appear to fight the Antichrist on the temple of the Mount which culminates in the destruction of the Jews and the second coming and the thousand year reign of Jesus Christ."? My only response to these saved people is extend my hand with money, point at my car and say, "Five dollars of Unleaded gas on pump two, please." How can anyone talk about eternity and really be *here*? Unless they don't want to take the responsibility of being here for others?

After I survived testicular cancer the first time, I returned to the Norwalk Hospital with flowers for the nurses who cared for me in radiation therapy. During the visit, I asked a crucifix-armed nurse about the kid who had brain cancer. She replied, "He's happier where he is now." I said nothing, but she infuriated me. That kid had dreams of being a photographer. He had his whole life ahead of him. *I know he'd never say that.* Then she added, "His mother didn't handle it well. I'm surprised. And she's a nurse. She should have known better."

I stared at this soulless stick figure with kneecaps supporting clueless hips and said, "Maybe she loved him."

So when I was diagnosed again with testicular cancer I was equipped with forgiveness and toleration to muffle and equalize the sounds coming from these benevolently misguided and over-modulated people. Not one of these pontificating Prayer Parishioners ever sacrificed their personal time or money to reduce my suffering. But if I recover they will be all smiles and jubilantly say, "I prayed for you! Our prayers were answered!" as if it validated their faith, as well as a pious way to nosily pry under my wound's scab to see if the ordeal converted me to their insensitive but compassionate beliefs. After surviving the first time, I'd have appreciated their concern for my welfare more if they had visited me once, or afterwards, flipped me a restaurant gift certificate or a bottle of wine to celebrate my cure. I didn't want to dilute my soul in my next cancer battle by enlisting false recruits who would flee at the first sign of personal commitment to defeat the enemy's advance and pray for me. I don't hold it against them. If they suddenly get ill or have a heart attack, I'll still give them a ride to the hospital, but I'll never come to see them.

Their Lord willing, of course. Or whoever or whatever comes first.

WHAT YOU MEAN, *WE* CHEMOSABI?

I**RANG IN THE NEW YEAR WITH CHEMOTHERAPY.** The only resolution I made was pressed between imaging scans. I stood in the hallway and stared above the doors at the signpost directing me to my Chemo-Centric World:

> Infusion Treatment Area
> Oncology Hematology BMT
> APHERESIS

I'm mentally everywhere today. Pick one: 1.) Washed up on the shores of another world with no survival skills. 2.) Bounced out of bounds by the jump ball of chance. 3.) At a *High Noon* showdown in a deserted street of an empty town, holstering nephrostomy bags, and strapped to get the draw on The Big C. I still end on the same plate: served up as a first course for infusion orientation:

Stanford Hospital Cancer Center Introduction to Chemo 001:

> **Course requirements:** Attendance is mandatory at the Infusion Center. Patient enrolls for 4 cycles of chemotherapy comprised of five straight days in sessions of 6 to 8 hours. Throughout each day, patient records their urine flow to ensure chemo hasn't shutdown kidney functions. After completing a cycle, patient has a chemo break of 2½ weeks to recover from infusion. During the break, the patient may be required to go through blood draws or transfusions, CT/PET-scans, surgery. Patient is expected to develop nausea, loss of taste, mouth sores, hair loss, blackouts, anemia, weight loss, fatigue, hearing loss, ear ringing. Patient is not required to dispose of their chemo bags, which are toxic poisons and are removed by HAZMAT (Hazardous Waste Materials crews.) **Cost:** Varies with your health insurance.

Daily Cycle Routine for Chemosabi's 6 – 8 hour day:

1.) Nurse takes vital signs. Patient ingests three anti-nausea pills: 80 mg. Emend, 24 mg. Zofran, 12 mg. Decadron.
2.) Receive a bag of a saline infusion to hydrate the body for the chemo. Patient also gets bag of 12.5g of Mannitol to encourage urination for chemo to pass quickly through kidneys to avoid collateral chemo-shutdown damage.
3.) After saline bag is completed, patient is shown a bag of Cisplatin 45 mg. in NS 250ml. Nurse checks your hospital bracelet, asks for your name and birth date, while another nurse holds chemo and verifies name on the bag. Data is entered on computer.
4.) After Cisplatin dose, another saline infusion is done because the two different chemo solutions cannot mix together.
5.) Second saline bag completed. Patient gets second chemo dose: etoposide 224 mg. in NS 500ml. Nurses repeat identification procedure.
6.) After etoposide, patient is flushed with saline solution.
7.) At the end of each session, nurse disconnects the IV from port, flushes heparin into port to prevent clotting, and tapes the six-inch Huber needle to patient's chest for treatment the next day. At the end of the week's cycle, nurse removes the Huber needle.
8.) Two-week-and-half week break between cycles to enable patient to recover from the effects of chemotherapy.
9.) After course completion, patient receives a PET/CT-scans to determine if tumor is gone.
10,) One month to recover then given an orchiectomy (Testicle removal.)
11.) Possible complex surgery to remove tumor from major artery.

After course completion, patient is required to schedule follow-up exams to ensure they are cancer-free. **Important:** Patient at admission signs a "consent" form absolving oncologist and hospital from any complications that result in your treatment (**Translation:** nothing is their fault, but if you don't sign the document you'll die. Man, even a car salesman gives you a better deal than this on a used car — well, maybe.).

IT WAS TIME TO CHECK-IN AND REGISTER MY COURSE OF ACTION. I stood at the Infusion doors. But I wasn't ready to step through the ropes into the ring. I search for a passerby in the second-floor hallway. It's 7:30 AM. I'm the only one here. No one is in sight. I stood near a poster of an old guy smiling with a golf club — obviously a survivor, but a genial old fart with a gut and a 7-iron slung over his shoulder who probably can't break 100 isn't exactly a motivating force to make me burst through the doors, belly up to the bar and order a round of chemo for the house. I took out a digital camera and waited, wondering if I should do this or not. I heard a person coming up the stairs. It was a young guy in a suit. Kinda a geek, attired in an outfit from the Single and Desperate Catalogue. He obviously worked somewhere in the hospital because he was healthy, smiling and obliviously running on his own power.

"Hi, would you take a picture of me?" I tentatively said. "I was diagnosed with cancer and—"

"Sure," quickly said the guy to deflect a long story.

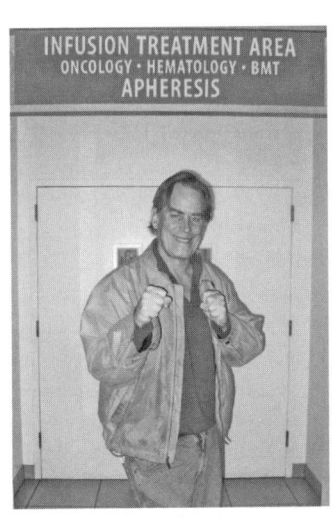

See infusion as a Fitness Gym to get stronger. Cancer doesn't have you. You have cancer. Do you know when you begin fighting cancer? When you agree to take the treatment! Some people can't face it and run. You chose to be here.

I assumed a boxer's pose in at the doors and said, "I have to show I'm going in to fight this. I'm coming out of here."

He snapped the picture. I thanked him, took the camera, and put it in my bag.

I turned and looked at the oncology sign, hung my head, and took a deep breath. There's an old joke where the Lone Ranger is surrounded by an Apache tribe and says to his Indian sidekick Tonto, "Looks like we're in trouble." Tonto replies, "What do you mean *we*, Kemo Sabe?" Now the joke acquired deeper meaning. I had a sudden edgy rush. The same vibe I'd get before I hit the stage to do stand-up comedy. I had to *perform*. You know when you really fight cancer? When you agree to take the treatment.

The doors closed behind me. It seemed like there was a suction and my life was sealed in a pressurized module. This was completely different than my first visit. Before I was a civilian. Now, I'm an enlisted recruit. The Infusion reception lounge is vacuum-sealed at room temperature. This isn't a waiting room. Everyone here is detached from Earth. We're passengers in a space station, drifting through the empty Chemo Galaxy. The caregivers are here with others but they're not *here*. We are the only ones *here*. It was quiet, like a wake. There's a somber heaviness in the air, as if I was being slowly lowered into an isolation tank filled with a thick numbing syrup. I walk softer and slower. My field of vision has shrunk. I'm on a voyage in another dimension. There are a few gloomy Chemosabis in knit caps, some wearing masks, aimlessly staring off. They slump in their chairs, silently suffering from the heavy gravity of their own presence. I'm not thin and have hair. But, I'm one of them now. I will not be like them. *I chose to be here!* I'm marching on this divot-pockmarked lunar surface, banging a big-ass bass drum and leading a parade of me. Watch me march, cancer. That's right, cancer, I'm coming for you!

"Good morning," I cheerfully address the receptionist. "How are you today?"

The woman is surprised by my greeting, sick patients rarely ask how hospital staffers are feeling. She said, "Very well. How are we today?"

"We're doing great. This is my first day of chemo. There is no other place I'd want to be. I'm here to get better," I said it loudly. I wanted other people to know I'm glad to be here. I hand her my Stanford patient identification card. "Here's my all-day ride pass." She also asks for a picture ID or a driver's license and if my insurance information is current. Then tells me to wait.

I cautiously angle myself into a cushioned chair that's bolted into the floor.

"Do you have a bad back?" asked a well-dressed woman in her sixties, seated near me. "I have a bad back from chemo treatments. I have lung cancer. I'm going through radiation too and they prop me up so it doesn't hurt, then I go into some heavy chemo. I was in remission for a while. It came back. It keeps moving."

I said, "I don't have a bad back." I bend over and slightly raise my shirt and show her my tubes. She isn't offended. "I have these tubes and when I sit down I have to be careful they don't catch on anything, otherwise I pull them out and I'll lose all my air and fly around this room like a loose balloon."

She laughed and wistfully said, "Ah, to have a sense of humor."

"With these tubes when I go to the bathroom I stretch them out like I'm curtseying. That's putting me way too much in touch with my feminine side." She laughed. "And the problem is I'm starting to like it." She weakly smiled.

I felt a vibrating hum in my pelvic region near the tumor. I thought, *Let the funny in me kill.* In stand-up, I killed rooms with funny. I'm no longer doing stand-up comedy. But I'm still funny. I have *that* power. Let the funny in me kill the malignant heckler trying to stop my performance. *Let funny kill.*

"I'm Fred. What's your name?"

"Miriam," she said.

"How long have you been coming to —"

"Seven years." She paused. "It keeps moving."

A nurse called her name.

She handed me her cup, "You can have my hot chocolate I haven't touched it."

"I'm not going to get cancer from it am I?" I replied, slightly recoiling. I take the cup and indignantly add, "What, no marshmallows?" Then I smirked.

"Ah, humor," Miriam longingly whispered, smiled and went to her treatment.

She'd been coming here for seven years. Seven years! Compared to Miriam, and so many others sitting by me, I'm a latchkey kid in chemo day care. I didn't feel fortunate. I felt humbled by these anthemic people from the country of courageous who don't need a breeze to proudly fly their flag.

A half hour later, my name is called. I take a deep breath and carry my gym bag, which holds my iPod and headphones, a biography of John F. Kennedy by Chris Matthews (I was still able to read at this stage.), lunch made by Laurie and juices (I could eat and didn't have mouth sores yet.), and an iPad a friend gave me. I'm in a room where they draw blood and administer chemo. There are two vacant recliners. No one is here but me and a male nurse. And I don't feel special.

"I'm so glad I have a port," I cheerfully said as I sat in a recliner. I pulled down the my shirt collar to show off the port above my right collarbone. "I couldn't hack having an IV in my arm all day."

"More people should have them." said the nurse, a black guy in his late thirties, cleaning the bump of skin that concealed my port. "For some reason oncologists aren't big on them and don't tell them."

"Maybe that's because oncologists never had an IV in their arm for eight hours."

"That's true, and doctors are the worst patients, believe me," added a passing oncology nurse.

"What's your name?"

The guy said, "Mars."

"Mars, huh? Now I know I'm officially on another planet."

A nurse walked by and said, "You're lucky, you have the best *stick* on the floor."

"Stick?"

"That's someone who is good at finding a vein. When they can't find one they usually look for me."

Mars spoke with a calm voice. He radiated a gentleness and concern. He unwrapped a package and took out a Huber needle, which is a thin clear tube about six inches long with a needle head on one end that inserts and locks into the port. On the other end is a connector where they can screw on test tubes, or a syringe as well as "access" an IV line to "introduce" chemo to my body.

"Ready?" Mars said. He pressed the needle head into my lidocaine-numbed skin and connected the power port with a click that sounded like buttoning up metal snaps on a jacket. "You're in business."

I laugh and said, "I felt nothing! I love my port."

"You keep this connection all week, then we'll remove it," said Mars securing the Huber needle's tube to my upper chest with tape. He flushed my port with a syringe of heperine to clear it, then drew blood and filled three test tubes.

"At least it's red."

"Yes, that is a good sign," he said, labeling the tubes.

"When I first came here I asked for a tour. I was depressed. I saw the people as powerless. I was wrong. I didn't see it the right way. I realized I had to rethink everything if I was going to get through this. Now when I see these recliners and the chemo, I see this place as a fitness gym, and the recliners with chemo are work-out machines, and I need to use them so I can get stronger."

Mars narrowed his eyes, studied me and said, "You have a great attitude. Some people don't. They have anger issues. One woman told me she was mad until she saw the children who had cancer then she felt better about herself."

I uttered in disbelief, "Children?" I paused. "What a sick selfish person. They don't see the pain in other people? I've had cancer before. All this suffering, if it doesn't connect you to the pain of others what is it?"

Mars shrugged and continued, "It's all anger issues. The five stages of grief. They're stuck on the second one. And they can't get past it: 'How could this happen to me? I didn't deserve this.'"

"I can't see it that way," I said. "Grief is a heavy thing. My Mom died from cancer. Dad died getting treated for cancer. When my Dad died that was harder than my Mom, because he was the last one. I was an orphan. I talked to Dad every day on the phone. But my grief became lighter and turned into the love my parents gave me. It made me stronger. Took awhile, but it did. Sometimes they visit me."

"Those things you say are true," he said.

"I have to tell you one thing. It's tough sitting on an exam table and having someone manhandle your last testicle like you're a horse at an auction. I mean, what can I say with my pants down on my ankles while a doctor is rolling my testicle? 'There's an extra $20 in this for you if you give me a happy ending.'?"

Mars smiled, compared the name on the stickers of the blood-filled test tubes with my hospital wrist bracelet and took my blood pressure.

"Your blood pressure is high," said Mars.

"Tell me about it. What's it, 150 something?"

"Yes."

"That's about right. When you go into this building you're going to work. When I go into a building that says 'Stanford Cancer Center,' that kinda has an effect of making my blood pressure go up more than if I'm entering a Chinese restaurant. Want to see my blood pressure lower? Take it when I'm at the beach."

"Yes, they call it 'white-lab-coat blood pressure.'"

I laugh.

Mars leaves my orbit. You have to respect a man who is his own planet. Especially when you don't feel you're on Earth and lost in space.

An oncology nurse introduces herself. Her name goes right through me. She is cordial. I follow her into the next room to start chemo.

She says, "Where would you like to sit? We have recliners, some with window views, but I think those are taken now. We also have side rooms with beds."

"No bed," I said firmly. "I'll sit in a chair. I will not lay down for cancer — ever."

I set up. I plug in an extension cord behind the recliner for my iPad, pull out headphones and iPod. I place my bag on the floor beside me so I can reach my book, and the juice, lunch and snacks Laurie packed for me each day. I felt chilly. I went into the bathroom and changed in my Farley surfboards sweatshirt. I wore it today for good luck. On my first day, I had to take the surf with me.

"Before I sit down, would you take a picture of me?"

"Sure."

I assume a surfing stance while holding the IV-pole.

"That looks good," said the nurse, snapping the shot.

I smiled and commented about my request, "What else you gonna do? Since I'm here I might as well build up my chemo fashion modeling portfolio."

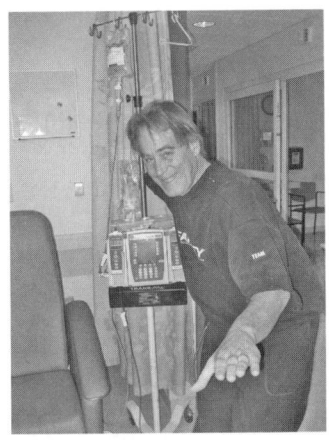

Surfing with my chemo IV-pole. I dubbed it my "Tower Of Power." Cancer is trying to close out my wave. I have to trim through the chemo foam to make it reach to the reforming curl of my life.

CANCER TREATMENT IS LIKE SURFING ACROSS A WAVE THAT SECTIONS. In surfing, "sections" means the wave breaks in front of you and reforms farther down the line. You have to skillfully angle your board and trim across the foam of the broken section to catch up to the reforming wave and surf it into the beach. Before I was diagnosed, I was riding a wave of life, tucked in the curl, but then The Big C sectioned and broke the wave in front of me. Now, I'm unsteadily driving through a chemical section of chemo, nausea, weakness, hair loss, lack of sleep, loss of taste and weight, blood transfusions, and more, hoping again to reconnect the reformed and unwrapping curl of my life. I made it across this section once before. Fred-27 finished radiation treatment and quit my newspaper job and lit out to California to do comedy and surf. I knew back then, if I strayed and didn't act on the opportunity, I'd lose the light of a reforming new life. We are all born with a pilot light. We have to be faithful to it. My pilot light is guiding me. I'm locked-in, totally committed within my tight pocket of retaliation, narrowly staying ahead of the cancer-chemo closeout. I've stayed true to my light. I've never strayed. It will get me through this section. It's become more than a beam. It's a force beyond. It's magnetically towing my soul. I'm driving through this foam, baptized by the approaching future I'm making of myself. It's all I got.

I'm ready for my chemo bake-off. I settle in the staging area of my infusion-station recliner. After 50 minutes of hydration, the nurse brings out a plastic pouch filled with a clear liquid. It's Cisplatin 45 mg. in NS 250ml.

"Is that chemo?" I ask, removing my headphones, leaning forward in the recliner.

"Yes."

"Can I *hold* it?" She hands me the chemo. I cradle it in my hand.

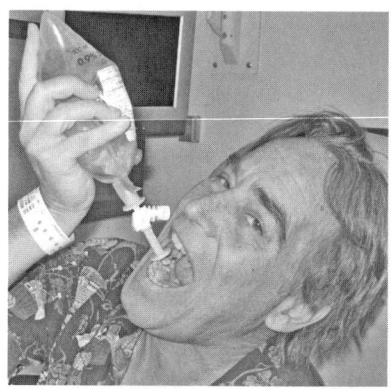

Bond with your chemo cocktail. Kiss the clear bota bag. Don't see chemo as a poison. Chemo's the *"Intravenous Energy Drink of Cancer-Free Champions!"*

I settle back into the recliner for lift off. The nurse hangs the chemo sack on my Tower of Power, which is my nickname for my chemo-draped IV-pole. The computer infusion pump clicks and hums like a Martian. I watch the clear Cisplatin cling then drip-drive its defoliant from a small plastic chamber to the tube into my port. Finally, it's starting! This is my hot landing zone. I'm pumped. After all the tests and consultations and scans I'm taking on the enemy at last! The Big C has been living inside me without permission. Multiplying and dividing and growing and spreading to look for blood sources because it has no heart, no circulatory system or bodily functions. My deadly opponent thrived in undiscovered darkness. It was a covert action. But now we're together at the Stanford Cancer Center, and I *know* it's hiding place. I imagine the mass as a slimy and blubbery, clear gooey bladder of pus-ripened nothingness. It's nestled in my healthy fruit-pulp like tissue. My stomach rumbles in the area where the nourishing tumor is cozily grazing and sipping away. The basking malignancy is unaware it's gradually being encircled. I imagine the chemo converging in waves, coating and singeing the tumor's shoreline, soaking and untangling its twisted strain's grip, tearing a fissure down its loathsome center core, breaking it apart so its rim crumbles, separates, slides and drops like a melting glacier in my warm bloodstream and floats to my kidneys where I will piss the dead cancer cells into the toilet, flushing it away from all that's good to where it truly belongs.

I watch chemo drip and say to myself, "This is as real as it gets."

As I slammed down my first boilermaker of chemo with a chaser of mannitol, I watched *Breaking Bad* on an iPad and listened to it on headphones. *Breaking Bad* is a noirish series about Walter White, a chemistry teacher who discovers he has cancer and decides to provide for his family by cooking crystal meth. What some people do to cover their deductible! I thought, this series achieves just the right touch of darkness to take the edge off chemo. Suddenly, my Spidey Sense detects a benevolently lurking presence near me. I see an attractive woman in her thirties cautiously trying to get my attention. She's dressed like she is going to a cocktail party — you know, nice skirt, make-up, jewelry, hair styled. I put *Breaking Bad* on pause, freezing a Mexican cartel member wielding a silver axe. I pull off my headphones.

"Yes?" I say, looking at her.

"Is this a good time for me?" she asks. Her tone is earnest and professionally calibrated to my situation. She smiles and nods a lot. She has a clipboard, folders and pamphlets. She smoothly introduces herself as a nutritionist who wants to create a diet plan for me to follow during chemotherapy. She pulls up a chair and runs through her skill-based support script. "Your taste buds are affected by chemotherapy. Most people experience a metallic taste in their mouth, so when you eat, use *plastic* utensils. Everyone who goes through chemotherapy reacts in different ways. Believe it or not, there are some people who actually *gain* weight."

"I wouldn't mind losing a few pounds," I said. "It will give me more float on my new board when I get back to surfing."

"And one day *you will*," she encouragingly said, but it was so urgently reflexive, she sounded insincere. "I have some literature here." Did she say "literature?" She wasn't handing me a novel. Her literature was a set of well-designed sheets entitled "Cancer Supportive Care Program" with pictures of enlightened and cheerful bald but healthy-looking people. She spouted her spiel like she was reading me a nursery rhyme as she stressed the importance of "forcing yourself to eat protein" and "drinking several 8-ounce glasses of water to increase fluid intake to flush chemo out of your system" and "eating small meals every couple hours." She benevolently smiled and starts riffing through the Chemo Specials of the Day on her recommended menu: yogurt, string cheese, applesauce in single-serving containers, raisins and other dried fruit, whole-wheat crackers, flavored rice cakes, unsalted nuts, baby carrots, low-fat cottage cheese, high-fiber cereal. She became more animated as she suggested ways to embellish these wholesome dishes. "*Good* olive oil with a squeeze of lemon juice perks up vegetables. Oh, add unprocessed wheat bran or flaxseed oils to cottage cheese. Mix frozen berries with low-fat yogurt — then maybe add some granola to create a fruit parfait, and also try yogurt toppings or spreads or dips with diced vegetables and seeds and nuts." This was a great diet if you were training for the Olympics — or a goat. Even when I was healthy, I rarely ate these foods. Outside of the fruit, yogurt, and pretzels, everything else she named was boring compared to a hot pastrami and swiss on rye with a big fat garlic pickle and a cold beer.

"You have to live day by day," unafflicted people benignly sermonize, as if this yawning-duh hymnal of perception passes for wisdom.

Living day-by-day? I don't have the luxury of days. I only have one day with thousands of dawns and sunsets. I do not have days. I have lingering moments interrupted by chemical warfare. And if I survive, I know it will always be one long day — forever. The best part about that, there's no such thing as the middle of the night. The time of day is just another numbered slot the ball of chance called my life drops into on a spinning roulette wheel.

You want to know where I am now? I'm walking down a long oblique corridor. Sometimes it gets angled, other times it drops like a trap door beneath me and forms a shaft where slide down its walls. Then it becomes a square hole that my round peg of life tries to squeeze through. While I'm walking in the corridor I hear the blunted murmuring of the outside world beyond my parallel shaft. People are securely moving along life's game board, rolling the dice of minutes and hours, laughing and discussing movies or TV shows and getting worked up over politics and making dinner reservations. They're safely lodged in weeks and years and bitching about work and griping about Mondays, pleased when it's hump day, and glad it's Friday, then make plans for the weekend and vacations and retirement. They are speaking a language I can't translate. Their preoccupations are a distraction, a trivial pursuit. At home, I hear a political show on TV where talking heads are ideologically barking about the Occupy Wall Street movement. I turn it off. I must leave the world of arguments to find my way out of here. I softly pad through this shock corridor on Novocaine feet. My passageway is gray, dimly lit along its top edge but ahead there is a light. I march to the veering light. This is a long march filled with suffering I sustain to prevail. I continue on this tough-love corridor, half smirking and repeating a Johnny Cash lyric to myself, "I fell in to a burning ring of fire." My laugh bleakly echoes hollowly down the hallway, but sounds ripe and full as it reaches the opening of light beyond me. I will get there. But until then, the corridor. Tentatively walking as steadily as I can on this spinning circular stage.

What's the worst that can happen, after the worst has happened? The Big C has me under siege. I'm disoriented in a recliner, drip-drying with chemo. I've been buried under a biological landfill of Comprehensive Metabolic Panels, HCG (Human Chorionic Gonadotropin), Systolic Diastolic, CBC (Complete Blood Count) with DIFF, LDH (Lactic Acid Dehydrogenase), Alpha Fetoprotein serums. Stung by a swarm of fine needle aspirations, blood draws, biopsies, labs and IV drips. My pelvic region has been declared a nuclear test zone for ultrasound, PET/CT scans. I'm snowballing in an avalanche of prescriptions for Lorazepam, Ondansetron Prochlorperazine, Beta. Ambien (Zolipidem), OxyCodone, acetaminophen, Percocet, docusate (Colace), Cephalexin. The clinical hazing centrifuge of procedures has broken me down

Today Cancer Tomorrow The World

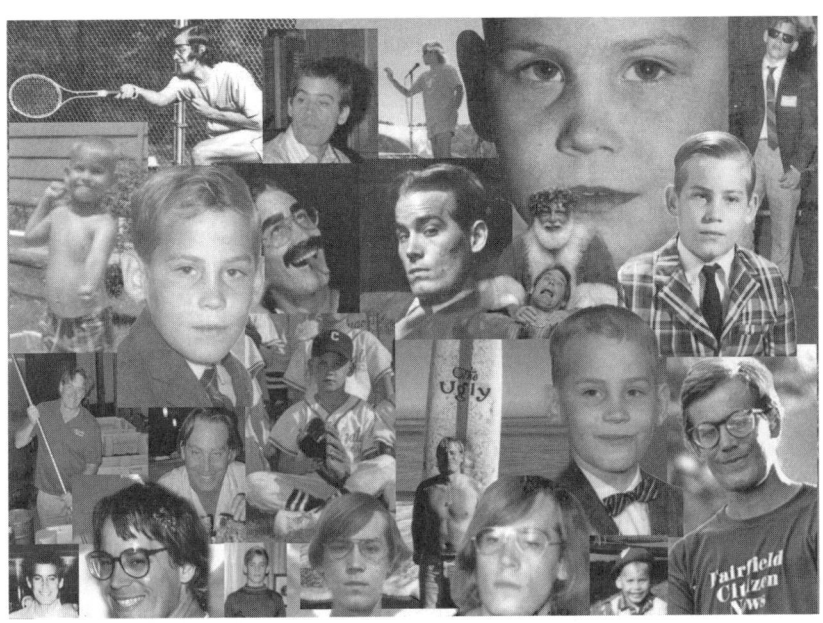

Your life is all you have to fight cancer. I'm 57. So I recruited 57 freds from every year in my life to join me in my battle. I had to multiply faster than cancer to divide and conquer. To save your life, you have to bring a life.

---

into blood levels of sodium, potassium, calcium, chloride, carbon dioxide, glucose, blood urea nitrogen, creatinine, protein, albumin, bilirubin, and liver enzymes. Doctors breed darkness at the speed of light. Port labs. No liquids or foods six hours before surgery. White and red blood cell counts. Pre-filled syringes with saline. Depot bags. I've taken so much heavy indoctrinating flak I was driven down by a spate of baseline marker numbers that stripped away my identity. I knew what I was but not *who* I was. This is my fault. I've made the mistake of allowing them to do reduce me to particles. Yes, I left The Me out of the process. I forgot about *my* life. I'm not a victim. *Cancer doesn't have me. I have cancer.* My life is all I have to battle against this disease. I need to take this fight to another level. I have to Occupy Fred! Cancer can only take life. It doesn't *have* a life of its own. I do! Does cancer have love, a wife, family, songs, friends, jokes, a surfboard? No, but I do! I'm 57. I have a fighting force of 57 Freds inside me! One from each year of my life. My souls outnumber the tumor's cancer strains. That counts in my favor. I sat in my chemo throne and closed my eyes and panhandle my past to hitch a ride back to the future. I issue a an S.O.S. casting-call to set the stage for all my Freds in the Theater of Me.

And here they come to help me kick cancer's ass.

"Guys, I need your help," I said to the mingling séance of me. "Fred-2: when his parents were asleep, snuck into the kitchen and poured flour on the floor. Oh, Fred-7: wearing the Mickey Mantle and Roger Maris M&M Boys T-shirt. Fred-13: got caught shoplifting at Britts Department store. Fred-18 who registered as a conscientious objector for the draft during the Vietnam War. Fred-22 — hey, rethink the puka shells and blow-drying your hair with mousse — it didn't look good then and it doesn't look good now. Fred-20, you streaked through the college cafeteria. Fred-29 who was a journalist strangled by a First Selectman candidate after the guy lost the election. Fred-32 who surfed. Fred-51 who harvested and made wine. Fred-34 who was an insult comic and said, 'I'm certain Jesus loves you, but in your case he's seeing other people.' Look at all you guys. No wonder I never amounted to anything." We laugh. "Okay Freds! Quiet down guys, I know you don't get along, but we have to stick together because we're all we've got. You all made me. Hey, you! The Fred over there. The one sulking and moody who feels no one understands him and believes the whole world is against him. Yeah, you, Fred-17. You're the one I need the most right now. You're the one who was molded from all the music from 1954–1972. You're the Fred who has the most immaturity, attitude, irresponsibility. No one can tell you anything! You have all the answers, don't you? You're the raw untamed Fred. The real juvenile rootstock unappreciative madness of me. The one who is a wiseass and kind of an asshole and all the Freds afterwards followed in your wake and felt guilty about your mistakes for years. There's Fred-13, who didn't want to be an illiterate moron after he realized he didn't know how to spell 'douche bag' on the bathroom wall — not exactly the aha moment of dense getting a clue. You started reading 'Quotable Quotes' in *Reader's Digest*. The quotes that struck you the most were Thoreau's on individuality. And that's when you read *Walden*. Thoreau used words and historic references that lead you to other books and the dictionary, and I expanded from there, reading other novelists, and responding to plays. It all began with the words: douche bag. Never underestimate a limited vocabulary. We need more than the Freds in this room to beat The Big C. Bring everyone else that you knew back then — friends, neighbors, relatives, and your toys, records, trading cards, favorite movies and comic books, magazines, but *don't forget the girls we loved.*" Then the girls and women arrived! Looking as young and beautiful as the first kiss they laid on me. The Freds danced with the girls and we fell in love again with each other and couldn't ever imagine we'd ever get into an argument. I admire the women's smiles and our joy of complete abandon. Oh, how I need you now, how I need your love. And here come people who *liked* me — friends and neighbors from every year of my life. And all my relatives, family. And most of all, Mom and Dad! Look at you! Young and in your first year of marriage. And Mom was pregnant with me. And I'm alive and kicking — always had to let people know I was around. Everyone, listen up. We have to overcome my limitations with the armed strength of our forevers to take down The Big C."

D raw strength from the music that inspired and still shapes you. Cancer can't rock. But **beware:** I've heard it likes rap. Crank up your volume. Cancer will never hear you coming!

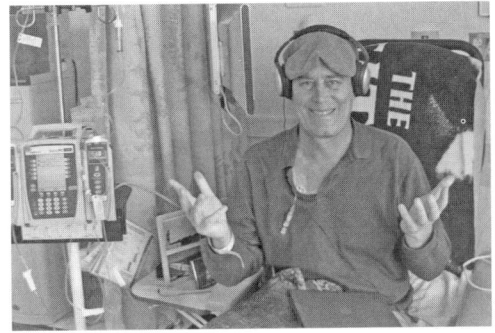

AND THE HITS KEEP ON COMING! What was the best way to shape all of the Freds and the years of my life into a fighting force? Music! I load an iPod with the sound check of my soul from every period in my life. I started with the music Fred-5 first heard coming from the green plastic grill of the radio my parents kept — for some odd reason — atop the refrigerator. There was *The Monster Mash* by Bobby "Boris" Pickett and *The Witch Doctor* by David Seville and *Mister Custer* by Larry Verne and *Mr. Bass Man* by Johnny Cymbal. When I was alone I pantomimed the songs and tried to do Bobby "Boris" Pickett going, "Whatever happened to my Transylvania twist?" And the warmth of all those Top 40 oldies from the '60s. It was like overfilling a flower pot and seeing the water get soaked up through the soil by the plant — mine is a dancing stem with strong and tightly green budded fists that rocks. I listen to all the tunes that inspired, animated and resuscitated all my Freds into a steady backbeat. Oh, what music! The Young Rascals, Turtles, Paul Revere and the Raiders, Four Seasons, Monkees, Sly and The Family Stone, Neil Diamond, The Association, Lou Christie, Petula Clark, Dave Clark Five, Johnny Rivers, Troggs, Guess Who, Mamas and Papas, The Grass Roots, Tommy James and the Shondells, James Brown, The Animals, all those girl groups, surf instrumentals, Simon and Garfunkle, Kinks, Beatles and Stones. When you go through high school that's the formative time when you dialed into all the songs on the AM-FM radio, every rock group, and all the cool albums. Humble Pie's *Shine On*, Led Zepplin's *Led Zepplin One & Two*, The Who's *Who's Next*, Chicago's *Chicago*, CSNY's *Déjà vu* and *Four-Way Street*, Credence's *Cosmos Factory*, Black Sabbath's *Black Sabbath*, Doors, Jethro Tull's *Aqualung*, the *Woodstock* soundtrack, Elton John's *Tumbleweed Connection*, Grand Funk Railroad's *Coming Home*, Steppenwolf's *Monster*. I left out Carole King's *Tapestry* — I only bought it back then because girls liked it. Songs I had heard hundreds of times outgrew and hadn't played in years like *American Pie* by Don McClean ("And as I watched him on the stage my hands were clenched in fits of rage. No angel born in hell could break that Satan's spell."). I was wounded. There was a war on. I had to hear that music again to heal. Over the years, I've accumulated tons of tunes. I'd like to have the ability to relax at the end of the day by pulling strings and licks on a guitar — but it's not me. I write, read, watch a movie or news. Then go off about it on the stage or radio. That's me. But I *listen* to music. I love it because it's something I can't do. When I was a teenager, my mother would say, "Aren't you tired of hearing that record?" But music requires digestion. I'd purchased a 45 and listen to it over and over again. Then move the needle to the last part of the song, listen to it, then put the needle in the middle of the song, then back to the beginning. That's when the tune became part of me. Every lyrical phrase and intonation, guitar lick, drum break and cymbal crash soaked into my consciousness and became me. It didn't matter if the music was before or after my time to send my troops into battle. But classical music didn't cut it. Clever and angry lyricists, folk, out-there jazz and rap didn't make the cut either. Droning, shoe-gazing alternative rock or electronica, another no. It had to have heart. It had to be fun. Beats I banged on the car dashboard while driving. A dynamic backing track that drew me out of myself to dance alone or with someone else! Surging music that made me feel alive every second! And I must be here every precious second! My playlist was stocked with the arsenal of bands to blow out cancer. Sleepy LaBeef, NRBQ, Bruce Springsteen, Howling Wolf, Dino, Al Green, Miles Davis, ABBA, Bee Gees, James Brown, Ramones, Duke Ellington, blues, British Invasion, Motown, rockabilly, doo wop, bad seventies music, disco, reggae, funk, eighties pop. I was fortifying a wall of sound and slamming together every note to defend myself against The Big C.

Some people are afraid to admitting their age by acknowledging the music that inspired them. They hesitate to make references that might reveal what's bottled up inside them is dated. I'm not dated. *I'm a vintage!* My contents are everything that comes before and after me. And if you can't keep up, get the hell out of the way. My Freds need leg room! Cancer doesn't have pipes, chops or licks. Cancer doesn't have soul. Cancer can't hear the music that propels my 57 Freds. The Big C will never see us coming!

I put on headphones, hit the iPod and launched our Fred counterattack with one of my favorite doo-wop songs, Randy and the Rainbows singing *Denise*.

> *Oh Denise, scooby-doo*
> *I'm in love with you, Denise scooby-doo*

The driving and foot-stomping and upbeat song of love creates a tingling force of climbing resilience inside me from the balls of my feet and buzzes through my spine and simmers along the sides of my skull and drives sound waves into the tumor and makes cancer feel pain for the first time in its absorbent lifeless mass.

> *Denise, Denise, oh, with your eyes so blue*
> *Denise, Denise, I've got a crush on you*

And who's joining the battle of me? Here come my gallant 57 doo-wopping Freds leading the charge! Followed by all those wonderful girls and neighbors and friends and surfboard-wielding buddies. Punching and kicking the beatless "large mass." Here come the rest of the reinforcements! Laurie, and there's Mom and Dad who returned from wherever they were to protect me once again. They are joined in the battle cry of this dance party of revenge by others I've forgotten who I touched somehow, plus all the memories that rise forth from the heart-beating notes of my human jukebox. A mosh pit of me closes in and shoves this malignant blob away from my healthy organs. It's Fredstocka-palooza!

> *Oh Denise, scooby-doo*
> *I'm in love with you, Denise scooby-doo*

The tumor sizzles along its mordant seams as if it's being cooked. Its screams are muffled within its deaden boneless, spineless cells. It squirms and shrinks and squeals like the square, hipless coward it truly is. My organs ripen and drive the power of rocking-ultrasonic-blue-note dreams against the force of a numb nightmare that can never be allowed to wake up.

"You're not taking us down," I snap. Tears roll and my fists clench, fingernails digging into my palms.

Cancer, I will dance on your grave while you die inside me.

> **Positron Emission Tomography (PET):** uses a camera and a radioactive chemical to look at organs to evaluate cancer. The tracer is a substance (such as glucose) that collects in cells using a lot of energy, such as cancer cells. A tracer liquid is put into a vein in your arm. Tracer moves and collects in the specific organ or tissue. The tracer gives off tiny positively charged particles (positrons). The camera records the positrons pictures on a computer. PET scan pictures do not show as much detail as CT-scans or magnetic resonance imaging (MRI) because the pictures show only the location of the tracer. The PET picture may be matched with those from a CT scan to get more detailed information about where the tracer is located.

I LOST MY BEARINGS. I was despondent. Why? I'm being dragged away by the riptide of prescribed circumstance. I know who I am but not where I am. I'm going through whenever a whatever is wherever. Resistance is futile. I must submit to the current's pull and hope when it finally releases my body I'll have enough energy to return to the destination of me. I was adrift with no sign of a shoreline. I had no clue how to get back. I was unable to touch bottom, struggling to keep my head above the sloshing chemo level of The Big C. Then a radiology technician slides me out on the tray from the cylindrical scanner's opening, as if he was pulling me from a wood-fired oven to see if I was done, or needed another five minutes. I came out baked, overcooked, blinking at the gleaming ceiling lights. I padded my pockets of consciousness and couldn't find the keys to start me. Or why I was. It didn't bother me. I was groggy, awakening.

"You were sleeping?" he said, stunned.

"Yeah, I've been beaten down all day, I have nothing left. I'm sapped."

"I'll have to do your head again. Your neck was bent. It'll take 10 to 12 minutes."

Now I remember, I'm undergoing a PET scan to see if cancer sprinkled my liver. Earlier they couldn't give me an effective scan because my kidneys were unable to process the contrasting dye. If The Big C's malignant smattering has spread, I'd spend five days in a hospital bed getting intensive chemo. I figured the worst was going to happen, because accepting its impact was less devastating if I *expected* it, than if I hoped it wasn't in my liver and was there. Weird, huh?

Four hours later, I was getting chemo. Nurse practitioner Nancy Quinn came up from the first floor of oncology. She's a sensitive, and pleasant lady, respectful. A professional who clearly enjoys her work, and understands the emotional gravity of each moment with a patient. Her face has slightly pinched wrinkles from years of softly delivering bad test results to patients. Those wrinkles are balanced out by sharp kindling eyes from years of healing. She is smiling, walking with a quick bounce. Her pupils are glowing with a crackling brightness.

She said, "Your results came in. Your liver is clean. I thought you'd like to know."

I SAT IN THE RECLINER AND THOUGHT ABOUT HALF-FILLED BOTTLES FLOATING IN THE OCEAN. Fred-12 fishing for flounder and crabbing with my Dad on a rowboat in Belmar Basin, New Jersey. I'd occasionally see discarded, half-filled bottles bobbing upright on the ocean's surface. I always wondered how long they'd last doing that before the bottles sunk. Later I made the connection between the bottles and people who remain economically afloat, half-filled with compromise, and the other half, an empty dream. I always vowed I'd never become of them. I always unfairly saw an enemy somewhere, I guess.

The adult world badgered me by asking, "What are you going to do with that?"

It was their standard response to my calling.

When I bought *Mad, Creepy, National Lampoon* and *Famous Monsters* magazines, rock and comedy albums, books...

"*What are you going to do with that?*"

When I majored in literature and theater in college...

"*What are you going to do with that?*"

When I decided to work at a winery...

"*What are you going to do with that?*"

When I did stand-up comedy...

"*What are you going to do with that?*"

When I took up surfing...

"*What are you going to do with that?*"

And now I'm getting chemo and sitting on a recliner. I'm jobless and near broke and saddled with debt from medical costs that if I repay will only get back to where I was before all this started — *and without my balls*. But I'll never apologize for my passions to the people who never lived up to theirs. They passively-aggressively cautioned me about all my choices, because they held their dreams in check with circuit breakers of false responsibilities. They can't gloat in the world of I-told-you-so because my dreams didn't die in my sleep. What happened to them? When the economy took a dump, they unfortunately lost their jobs and retirement and are running through their 401ks because they can't afford to sell their homes which have dropped in value. And on top of that, they can still end up *here* too. Some do. I want to say to them, "What are you going to do with that?" But don't.

I believe the life I *built* gives me an edge most people don't have. I never used anyone to advance myself or came out ahead on a business deal at the expense of someone else. I never left with more than I gave. Any time I took a chance or made a career change, my friends supported me, but people who I thought were my friends, under the guise of concern, always said, "What if it doesn't work out?" They were half-filled beer bottles too. You need the commitment to have nothing to fall back on but yourself. If you time it right, it's not such a bad a drop. I kinda like the sound. I didn't want to be half-fulfilled. Hope swallowed my contents. Full is the fuel of my dreams. Cancer can't drain me.

FLUSHED OUT THE END OF THE WEEK BY FIRST CYCLE OF CHEMO, I exit the Infusion Treatment Area sluiced with toxic-healing chemicals. I go downstairs. My body percolates with the aftertaste of chemo bisque and meds. This hangover feels like my brain has been turned into a damp towel left inside a gym locker for five days. In two-and-a-half weeks, I'll begin the second of my four cycles. How do you call sitting in a recliner for eight solid hours and getting chemo dripped through a tube in your vein a *cycle*? I lean toward calling it an Inner Ring of Hell — but I can't bring myself to completely believe that. I cling to the conviction that all this heaviness and pain is curing me, and I'm chemo-concentrically spinning *away* from an Inner Hell. *Chemo: The UnderLord Of The Rings.*

I wearily sit downstairs in the hospital lobby and wait for a friend to pick me up. I definitely didn't have enough mental focus to drive myself. A doctor told me chemo patients who drove to their treatments frequently got into accidents on the hospital grounds; in fact, security was told if there was an accident and the person was bald to call the hospital not the police. In front of me was a table with old magazines, addresses of subscribers torn from the covers. I picked up a *New Yorker* but couldn't focus on the prose. My ashen brain cells were tapped out. I glanced at the cartoons. Yeah, I remember the world of funny, I thought, nodding and not laughing. Nearby, a volunteer played the piano. At least it wasn't the goddamn harp! The pianist occasionally hit a few wrong notes of

What a Wonderful World that echoed into the vaulted ceiling. I glanced up from the magazine and took in the procession of fellow refugees driven from the World of Health who were entering and leaving the hospital. Old people hobbled on walkers. Others were pushed in wheelchairs, dejectedly hanging their heads and staring at their scuffed slippers. Shuffling Chemosabis with face masks, wearing drawstring sweat pants. Then I recognized a woman in her early thirties with her husband. They were with two children. She was a fellow Chemosabis. We had a nodding acquaintance when I wheeled my mighty Tower of Power by her recliner to drain my bags in the bathroom.

"I noticed you had a port too," I said, smiling. "My name is Fred."

"I'm Barb," she said, shaking my hand. She looked tired. Her husband had a worn face as he was trying to rein in their energetic little kids, who were circling and pleading to get candy at the pharmacy. The parents were anchored in sorrow, but their children clearly had no clue to how sick their mom was.

I put down the magazine and said, "This was my first week."

Barb commented, "I've been doing this a long time. And mine is inoperable. So they chemo me wherever they find it. To contain it. This has been going on for years. If you have trouble eating, the protein drinks are good for you, but most of them taste awful. The Carnation Instant Breakfasts are real good. Be sure to take your anti-nausea medicines at home, even if you don't feel nauseous. Burping is a warning signs you might throw up." Her husband glanced at her. It was time to go. If you didn't know she had cancer and he was a caregiver, you'd simply assume they were exhausted parents. Then she gave me the best advice about chemo, "When you're done, don't take this place with you. When you're home don't think about coming here. Only think about what's around you. Don't be hard on yourself. Give yourself a break."

So many Chemosabis and caregivers I met were suffering, but they never complained or asked for sympathy, they simply described their situation, and always tried to relieve the pain of others by giving them advice based on their experience. So far, most of the doctors I dealt with hadn't acquired that skill.

I watched the family leave, wondering if Barb was going to make it. If she died, would her children regret years from now what they *could* have said to her? They were too young to understand anything except themselves. Oddly, I backtrack to the past and remember Dad's green leather barcalounger in the family room of our Freehold, NJ home. Fred-11 inexplicably liked the snapping sound a ballpoint pen made when I stuck and poked it through the leather chair's arm. My father was furious when he saw ten tiny round holes in the expensive chair. He called a meeting with my two sisters, brother, and myself and demanded to know who poked holes in the barcalounger. I said nothing. As we got older, he'd occasionally make a reference to the incident and grunt, "Another mystery." Years later, grief-stricken Fred-55, sat beside Dad's hospital bed. He was dying, and I still couldn't bring myself to confess I stabbed the barcalounger.

WHERE HEADS HAVE NO PART

MY HAIR NO LONGER FELT LIKE MINE. It resembled monofilament fishing line pasted to my head. During my first cycle of chemo, I examined my reflection to detect signs of balding. My hair only looked flatter. Then one day, I ran a comb through my hair and tugged out a gnarled nest. It's happening, I'm losing it, I thought. It's like watching myself peel away and melt. I didn't want to see flesh streaks between thinning hair that resembled strips of bacon on my head. I knew how ridiculous guys looked with comb overs. When I was told I'd lose my hair from chemo, I was upset. It was like scalping my personality. But, if I wanted to get through cancer's battlefield, I couldn't afford to remain attached to the way I once looked. A full head of hair belonged to the healthy — it had nothing to do being deployed to fight against The Big C. If I clung to hair, I'd be in denial. I had to let that Fred go. Instead of being resigned, I anticipated and *accepted* my fate. Chemo was a *choice* I made. *I had to take control.* I needed to retrofit a combat-ready look and wear a different uniform to survive. I had to soldier on. I decided to shave my head.

I called Maggie McReynolds, who always cut my hair. Maggie is a feisty lady who also does a lot of volunteer work and has driven me as well as many others to chemotherapy. She came to our house and shaved my head for free. Laurie and Maggie's husband Phil stood in the kitchen to watch my shearing.

I asked Maggie to do the sides first to see how I looked in a Mohawk, then said."If I surfed looking like this I'd get waves because everyone would fear me."

The next morning Shaved Head Fred prepared to leave at 6 A.M. for chemo. I inspected myself in the mirror. My scalp looked like a heavily peppered pink Easter egg. There were miniscule fleshy spots where chemo had burned out hair. Bald didn't bother me now. In boot camp, the military shaves your head to humiliate and dehumanize you into a killing machine for war. I was drafted and processed at the Chemo Induction Center to prevent The Big C from invading my home turf. I shaved my head to *retain* my humanity and become a new breed of fighter: a conscientious objector who wants to kill. I'm heading out to reclaim occupied territory in a land where peoples' heads have no part.

CLUMPS OF YOUR HAIR WILL FALL INTO YOU HANDS.

Take control! Get your head shaved. Have fun with it. See how you look in a Mohawk. Now, you're inducted to fight The Big C. You don't need a wig! Wigs are for wussies! Be proud of your armored Chemo Skin Head. It's your combat uniform. You've *accepted* the battle. It's crunch time. And while you're at it, dude, get yourself a cool hat.

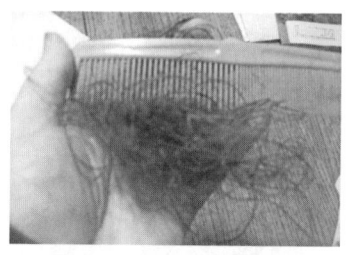

You *possess* two powers Cancer can't defeat.

You got…

Soul
&
Style!

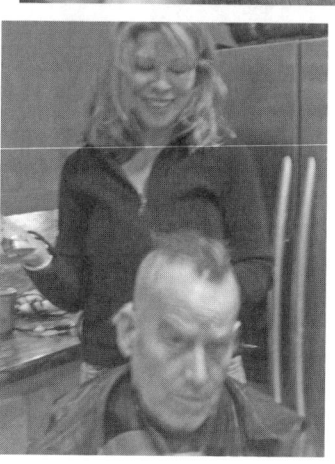

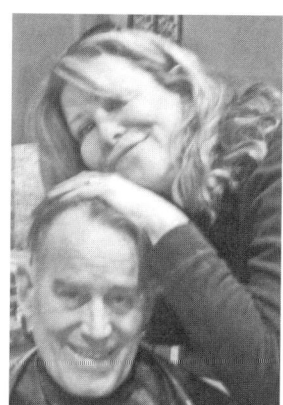

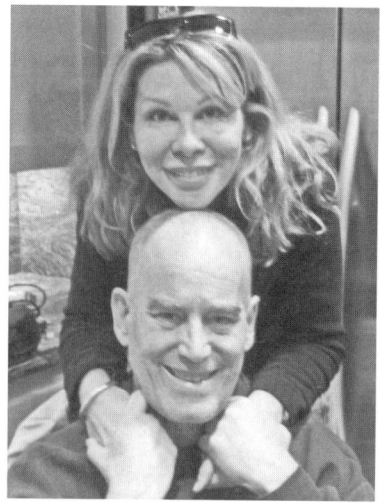

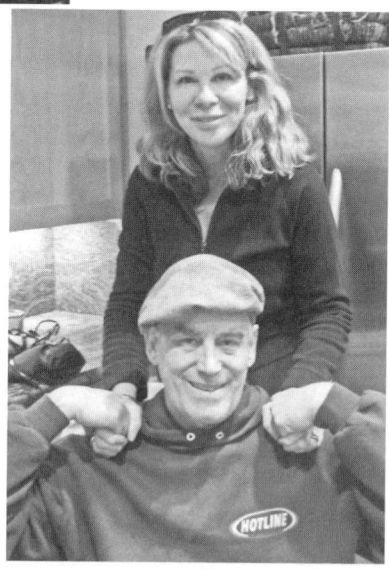

When you're on the infusion fashion model runway, don't dress like a typical dreary chemo dweller or people will think you're suspect taking a perp walk without a cop. It's a great look if you want to be remanded into custody.

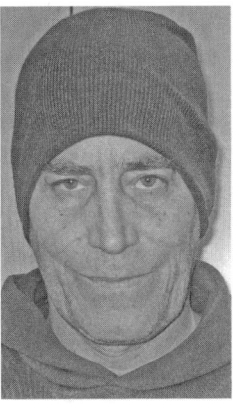

I REFUSED TO CONCEAL MY BALDNESS UNDER A STANDARD-ISSUE KNIT CAP PULLED DOWN ABOVE MY EYES. I wasn't going to be a sullen Chemosabi. I'd wear a knit cap at home. It's the best way to keep my head warm. But I took an oath to never wear a knit cap getting chemo or out in public.

Why? Well, for the following reasons:

DURING CHEMO IF YOU WEAR A KNIT CAP IN PUBLIC YOU'LL HAVE THESE SIDE EFFECTS:

- Begin to think rap music isn't that bad.
- Hand out pamphlets depicting 'The Way.'
- Buy a large wooden instrument that makes unpleasant sounds and practice playing it at organic farmer's markets by the artichoke section.
- Manage a recycling center.
- Drive a beat-up truck that has 'Firewood for sale' sign on it.
- Hang at skateboard parks or construction sites, be surly, and smoke. Actually, hang anywhere, be surly and smoke.
- Say the phrase, "I'm sorry, we don't have that part in stock."
- Change my name to Baga Vad-Vishnu.
- Get mistaken for a crossbow mentor.
- Stand in front of restaurants and valet park cars.
- Believe you resemble a sous-chef at a homeless center.
- Introduce yourself as a person who isn't from the future, but has no future.
- Pursue a career modeling camouflage clothing for Survivalist publications.
- Stand by a barrel of burning wood until the Dockworkers strike is solved.
- Tell people you're a State Park Lighthouse Docent.
- Think drawstring pants are bling.
- If you're near kids, people check your ankle for a parolee tracking device.
- Show up unannounced for warehouse job interviews.
- Claim you're one of the original *Z Boys from Dogtown*.
- Hope your jail sentence is reduced because you were in an Outreach program.

If you have to chemo, go with a flare. Be bigger than the moment. Dress like you don't need chemo. Chemo needs you. But I admit, wearing a beret made me want to do two things: 1.) See foreign films with subtitles. 2.) Hang out in coffee shops and make pretentious comments about current events or people I didn't know.

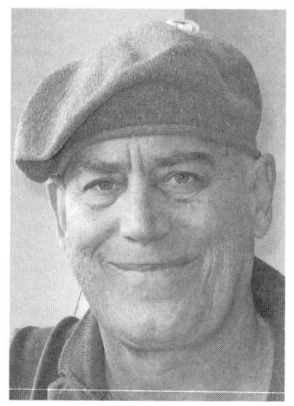

So, weeks before I began chemo, I did an un-guy like thing: I accessorized. I shopped for Chemo-Fashion flare. I purchased a cool looking light blue hat that flopped at a rather rakish angle. It resembled a Special Forces beret, and in a way it was. Most of the downtrodden Chemosabis wore drawstring pants, sweatshirt and a knit cap pulled low on their faces. They looked like cancer captured and had taken them prisoner. That was surrendering to cancer — or worse, to current fashion. I vowed that no matter how bad I felt, I'd dress up and stride with style into the Infusion Treatment Area. I thought back to the source of my clothing inspiration. When Fred-24 took a lunch break in Bryant Park behind the New York Public Library, I started talking to a retired guy on a bench, who gave me the best way to prepare for a job interview: "Dress like you don't need the job." I'm sure that retired man in the park probably has no idea how far his advice carried me. I decided to dress like I *didn't need* chemo.

FRED-30 WAS PERFORMING STAND-UP COMEDY ON AN OPEN-MIKE NIGHT AT A BIKER BAR IN BELMONT, CA. The regulars were mad because they couldn't play liar's dice or shoot pool during the show. A misspelled sign at the bar said "Knives must be *sheethed*." I stood on a warped stage flat. The mic picked up feedback from the PA System placed beside it. I was telling tattoo jokes.

"I'll show you a tattoo," growled a drunk burly biker, who had a gray ponytail, T-shirt, leather vest, torn jeans, and attached to his belt was a chain running through his wallet. He stepped on the stage, pulled down his lower lip, and said, "Tell them what it says." Inscribed in his inner lip were the words: "Eat Pussy."

I turned to the audience and stated, "Your tattoo says: 'Open other end.'"

A huge laugh from the crowd.

I wondered, where did that line come from?

And here I was in another stage, The Big C has pulled down my lip and looked down inside me.

My life is a performance. And the kid *needs* a comeback.

AFTER ADJUSTING THE NEPHROSTOMY TUBES AND MY DRAINAGE BAGS, I sat on the toilet in our bathroom, assuming a semi-constipated pose to "void" my bowels. I feel like I'm attempting to blow a lead balloon out of my ass. Forcing a bowel movement is how some people get a heart attack and die. The cause of death is "obstruction because of a large mass." When I was Fred-25, I was making my Town Hall rounds as a reporter for the *Fairfield Citizen-News*, routinely checking agendas, land transfers, and certificates of death. I found a typing mistake describing an 87-year old woman's COD as: "obstruction due to a large *ass.*" I showed it to a clerk, who replied, "I'll change it, but you know what? It's *true.*" What an exit strategy. Have cancer but die taking a dump! What's next? Starting my day with a stool-softener omelet? I laugh at myself. Anyway, I'm exhausted, crouched and ready to take the snap. I look to my right. I'm not alone. Hunched in the nearby litter box is our cat Groucho, a devious Maine Coon. He's staring at me and voiding too. I wonder if Groucho and I are performing a different kind of "synchronized cycling." He's named Groucho because he has a Groucho-Marx like fur mustache pattern under his nose. Groucho is one of our three rescued cats. The other two are Brooksie (Given to us by a rocker Greg Kihn who admired the Baltimore Oriole's third baseman Brooks Robinson.) and Bogie (After Humphrey Bogart.). While Groucho and I are bowel cycling, Bogie jumps onto the sink counter. I know what he wants. I turn on the water so Bogie can drink from the tap. Brooksie enters and brushes against my ankles, looks up at me, and expects his morning pets. I scratch his spine just above his tail. He turns and licks my knuckles with a rough tongue.

Our cats provide love below our knees. The cats don't live with us, they *allow us* to live with them. They sense I'm out of sync and try to comfort me. The cats are a combination support group and Axis of Evil. Why Axis of Evil? Because if I'm relieving myself or stepping out of the shower, they instinctively target and whack the tubes dangling out of my back.

Great, it's bad enough I have cancer. Now, I'm a living cat toy.

IF LIFE IS A DREAM THEN DEATH IS A WAKE-UP CALL. Don't kid yourself. Life is as real as it gets. Good health enables you to deceive yourself that life's a dream. You can only unspool a dream cord if you fought for the promising life your parents envisioned for you when they first held you in their protective arms so you could reach out with tiny hands through a blurry dark void and grasp their fingers to launch yourself into this world like a trapeze artist working without a net, hoping that somewhere ahead there's a swing to grab and prevent your fall…then, you're living the dream. In the darkness that exists within the bright hospital lights, I cling to a swaying hope above the oblivious healthy ones and dreamless sleepwalkers of a wide-eyed reality.

What builds your foundation are the people who constructed your life when you weren't aware of it. All the personal flaws you fought against to keep the dream machine of your heart-pulsating fingertips reaching, grasping, and hugging—climbing. And keeping your eyes open wide because you are emotionally within every moment and struggling to carve your style in spite of the practical demands of the world and the disappointments in your quest to succeed as yourself. And all the time believing there is something unique inside you that you still haven't truly articulated just yet. They say there's nothing new under the sun but there's a shitload happening *above* the sun.

FRED-15 HAD A BOSS HO-SCALE RACING SLOT-CAR LAYOUT IN THE BASEMENT. I designed the track around papier mâché mountains on a sheet of green-painted plywood, which I positioned atop the ping-pong table. My buddies and I raced cars, while we drank cokes and ate potato chips. It was a tricky course with straight-aways ending in tight turns, so if you gunned it too fast, your car would sail off the raceway onto the concrete floor. While I wound my Aurora slot car on the track, enjoying the drive through my miniature world, I imagined the day I'd be in a car cruising along in the real world.

Now, I'm winding through the tight turns of cancer's tightly binding speedway. For brief and unpredictable intervals, I'm tentatively freed from chemo's remote-control effects. I put the pedal to the metal powered by the only fuel I have: scattered scenic views of my life. I'm no longer gripping a remote control. For a moment, my steering ability isn't restricted by a guide pin in a slot. But, this is as real as it gets. I remain humble and stay the course, otherwise I fall off its edge.

In the World of Cancer the Earth is flat.

CHEMO AND I ARE TUMOR HUNTING. I draw the bow of my life-forming core and slowly attempt to precisely focus the heartlessness of The Big C into the center of my living longitude and latitude crosshairs:

> **PAST LONGITUDE (JANUARY, 1968):** Winter in Freehold, New Jersey. 8 A.M. Fred-13 lying in bed. A dark morning. The blankets pressing heavily upon me, weighing me down with warmth. Mom and Dad's comforting voices downstairs in the kitchen. The sizzling of kielbasa cooking. I hear the flaring furnace through the wall's heating vents. My two sisters stirring in their room. My little brother asleep in his. I look outside. A small bank of snow has sifted between the storm and interior window. Howling winds sprinkle sizzling hisses of shifting sharp crystal flakes like salt across the white desert of snow-encrusted streets. Icicles hang like stalactites along the rain gutter, as if I'm peering out a cave not a room. The falling snow storm is illuminated by the streetlights along Stonehurst Boulevard in front of our home. Not one flake of a chilling world touched me.

PRESENT LATITUDE (JANUARY, 2012): Winter in Palo, Alto, California. 9 A.M. Fred-57 in a recliner getting chemo from his Tower of Power. A gray morning. I gently turn my hips to create slack in the nephrostomy tubes so they won't tug the catheter wires stuck in my back. Rain pelts and winds rattle the Infusion Treatment Area windows. Moist raindrops blend their glass-beaded backdrop into the trickling steady direct-to-consumer drop by drop cancer defoliant fluid monitored by the IV tube's drip chamber. I stare but I'm not here. I'm clutching a smile and swooping into the present powered by the gravity of the past from my Freehold bedroom, remembering the snow flakes floating down the illuminated streetlight beams and gradually packing its covering over the outside world as I drift under heavy covers of memory for protection against a chill factor swirling *inside* this room.

I can only broadcast myself with transmissions that formed within me. Where the personality of life had an intense armored momentum, an attacking force of an established presence to strangle cancer. Guided by Longitude-1968 and Latitude-2012 coordinates, my life anchors a pivoting point to home in my pelvic realm on the Big C. I'm trying to drive back its malignant advance. On my tissued tundra, I'm tracking the lumbering mass with the drawn bow of my life. I step cautiously. The wilderness here is full of mutations. Ahead I can make out the swirling clear tumor distorting my surroundings. I see through the tumor's deceptive clarity. It's an inanimate thing that has a cancer motion within it. I'm digging my feet into my soft and unsteady organs, tightening the bow, aiming deep with the sight pins into the kill zone where the tumor ripples, spirals out and spreads. My smile pulling the weighted bowstring drawn back by the embrace of the mother and father who raised me. And I think of the first joys of arriving in California and stepping on the stage to do stand-up and making my own wine and surfing waves and cracking the mic open on radio and falling in love and how broadening out with strong friendships has risen to enliven and embolden me against this nothingness that's unable to camouflage itself against me because no one will give it cover — that's cancer's weakness, it doesn't have a life, it can only live through others. No one loves a user. I release the tight smile of my drawn bow and fire all of me and follow the shaft of my light beam as its pointed lance wetly snaps into the moist binding swirl of The Big C, splattering its slurping curving center, as if like I shot into a pool of gunk. It shivers with useless spinelessness and gets swallowed up in its own backwash and a glow bursts within its core.

Direct hit. Cancer skulks back in the shadows. Squeal and shrink you wonder of deathlessness.

I sit like a decoy in the recliner to draw my nemesis out for another clear shot, safe in my sniper's nest — sighted, aiming and primed to drop The Big C. *I'm not moving but I'm coming to get you.* We're in this together.

"**You live in a dream world.**" I've heard it my whole life. From teachers. From drinkers of lost dreams. From people chained to their medical and dental benefits at their particle-board desks who never tore off their day-job costume to find the superhero within themselves and fly away. "Mr. Reiss, you live in a dream world," they'd sternly say, getting ready to lecture me on my way of life. On the plus side, if they're right and I do live in a dream world, when I wake up, they'll be gone. And so will cancer. What will those two do without me?

I guess they'll always have each other.

Cancer is the ultimate zen master. There are people who want to achieve enlightenment and "live in the moment to appreciate every aspect of life through actualizing the awakening of everything's wholeness and interconnectedness by losing their attachment to who they are so they can bear witness to life around them and become it."

As I watch chemo seem to precipitate in the drip chamber of an iv-tube, I know a gyre of cancer is "actualizing the awakening" of a tumor into the "wholeness" of a malignant burl "living in a moment of inter-connectedness" to my cells and I've lost my attachment to who I am but *I don't want to become it*.

When you have cancer, zen is assisted-living for the healthy.

Cancer reminded me of a guy named Cousey. Fred-7 in Clifton, New Jersey, came running back to me. Cousey was a bully in our neighborhood. He was Cousey-12. He was the first kid I knew who said "fuck" and "shit," and hawked and spit mucous — those were the only impressive things about him. If Cousey saw us kneeling on a curb and flipping baseball cards against a wall, he'd snatch our cards, rip them up and laugh. He'd always pick fights with me. He'd pin me, put his knees on my chest, and hawk up mucous and dribble and dangle a string of salivated drooled goo above my face. I'd squirm and turn my head from side to side. Cousey wanted me to give up. He'd grunt, "Reiss, you *give*?" I never would. He'd lose interest, get off me, then make some crack like, "Let the baby have his bottle." One time, I struggled up, grabbed a big rock and threw it Cousey. I just missed his head. I thought he was going to kick my ass. He didn't. I think it was because he knew even if he did beat me up, I'd throw another rock at him — maybe a *bigger* one.

Cancer deeply digs its knees into my chest. It's trying to work up spit. My lips clench and pucker. Tears flow. But I'm not squirming. I'm not turning my head. Cancer can hawk up and dangle its dark goo over my face, but it's not touching me. I'm defiantly staring down the worst cancer can do to me and feeling the ground around me for a rock. *I'm not giving.* You hear me? *I'm not giving.*

A Title Match at The Infusion Grand Arena

THE CHEMO KID
vs
THE BIG C
The Showdown of a Lifetime

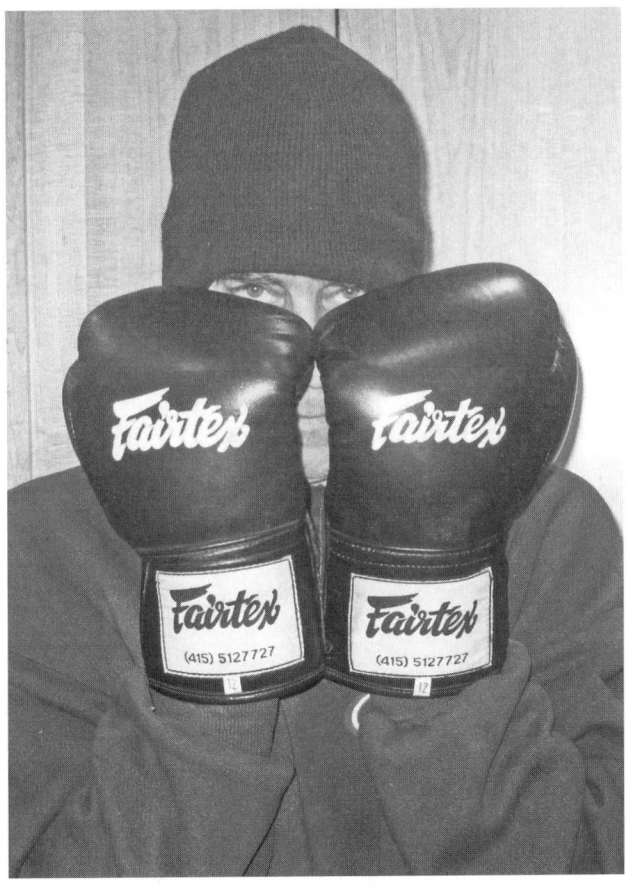

ROUND ONE I'M STANDING IN THE BOXING RING'S CORNER, SUPPORTING MYSELF WITH MY TOWER OF POWER. I don't look like a strong contender. I'm bald. My hair clippings are on the floor at my feet. Catheters in my back. Urine filling the depot bags strapped to my legs. I'm cold. The house lights illuminate the ring. The arena is dark. So far, no spectators.

"Ladies and gentlemen, welcome to the main event," said the ring commentator. "In this corner, wearing a blue hospital gown, vital signs: Blood pressure 142/93. Pulse: 76. Temperature: 97.2. Respiration 16, and weighing in at 229, the challenger, originally hailing from Freehold New Jersey, The Chemo Kid. And in the opposite corner, in blood-red trunks, from the challenger's pelvic region, undefeated in his last 55 infusion bouts, The Big C! In this rematch there is no standing-eight count, there's no three-knockdown rule in effect, no TKOs, no neutral corner, no referee. There's only rule in this title fight: *only one survives!*"

The Big C dances into the center ring, taunting me by pounding his crimson gloves together. His movements are clunky and powerful. He's growing. His arms adorned with the hospital identification bracelets of vanquished challengers.

I shuffle to my foe, wheeling my durable aluminum 5-foot high Tower of Power on casters, a chemo bag sways on the pole's curved hook as a tube dangles down to the medical port above my collarbone. I'm too weak from chemo to raise my gloves.

We stand face to face and have our stare down in the center ring.

The Big C's face is concealed by a brown square hood of sticky fabric. The burlap-like mask has no openings. His breathing draws the hood's gauze into the shape of a concave circle that bellies in and out with a moist crinkling sound. I thought he'd be darker. His skin is transparent. I can see into his body. The malignant champion's metastasizing muscles are a translucent silver liquid of tiny kidney-shaped nodules. He has only one organ. In the center of his chest is a throbbing grayish blob. It's the shape of the mass I saw in my CT scan.

My tumor is his heart!

The Big C doesn't speak. He doesn't have to. He's a hitter.

We return to our corners.

A bell clangs to start My First Cycle of Chemo.

The ringside commentator launches into the play-by-play, "The Big C is an unorthodox fighter. That doesn't bother him. He says let it bother *the other guy*. These two faced each other in the ring 30 years ago. Since then the champ has tuned-up in fight after fight, establishing a string of knockouts. The Big C comes out strong and lands a right. Letting The Kid know who the bigger man is. The challenger certainly doesn't belong in the same class or ring. The Chemo Kid has his arms at his waist. He has no concept of a counterpunch, showing no speed. Hard left and right shots nail the challenger and the champ lets loose with a flurry of jabs. The Big C is looking to air this out in the first round."

I've got nothing. I'm drained by chemo. I'm nauseous. I take the beating. Going through this brutal chemo-cancer match means early on, I'm going to get tagged with more punches then I throw, but I believe every blow I'm taking is somehow weakening The Big C. *I have to*. It's all I got.

"The champ is in total command. Throwing every shot with murderous intent. Oh! A hard overhand right. Boom! Rung The Chemo Kid's bell with that one!

The champ is pouring it on. A right, a left, again lands a right! He's picking The Kid apart. This can't go on. This is what we're talking about when a guy comes up against a real champion and goes against that talent. How can The Kid absorb such punishment? The Big C continues to pummel The Kid. He's trying to put him away. The Kid is walking straight into these blows. Oh! A body shot. Right hand, left jab. Vertigo. Next stop Queer Street. The Chemo Kid is on the ropes. Look at his eyes. He doesn't know what clinic he's in."

A bell clangs several times to end the round.

The ringside commentator says, "The Kid is still standing. The Big C looks confused. In past fights, his opponents have dropped in the first round. But the challenger is still standing! What's holding him up?"

"Is that all you got?" I weakly blurt, coughing, buckled over, deeply fatigued and bracing myself on the Tower of Power's steel pole.

I look into The Big C's see-through chest at my throbbing tumor: there's a fizzling around its edges, a thin gray stream is seeping out of its knotted mass into his clear body, streaking out a slow stain.

I'm starting to metastasizing into him.

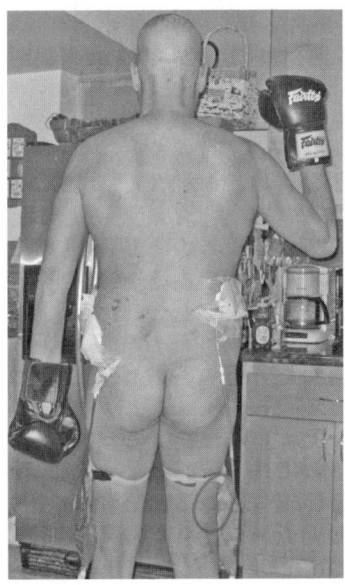

People recoiled in revulsion at the catheters and tubes in my back. The bags are the knapsack I need to climb to the summit. The tubes are ropes to pull myself out from the tunnel of darkness into the light. Look for the fight in me. I'm not ashamed! I'm *proud* of my body armor because I'm fighting for my life.

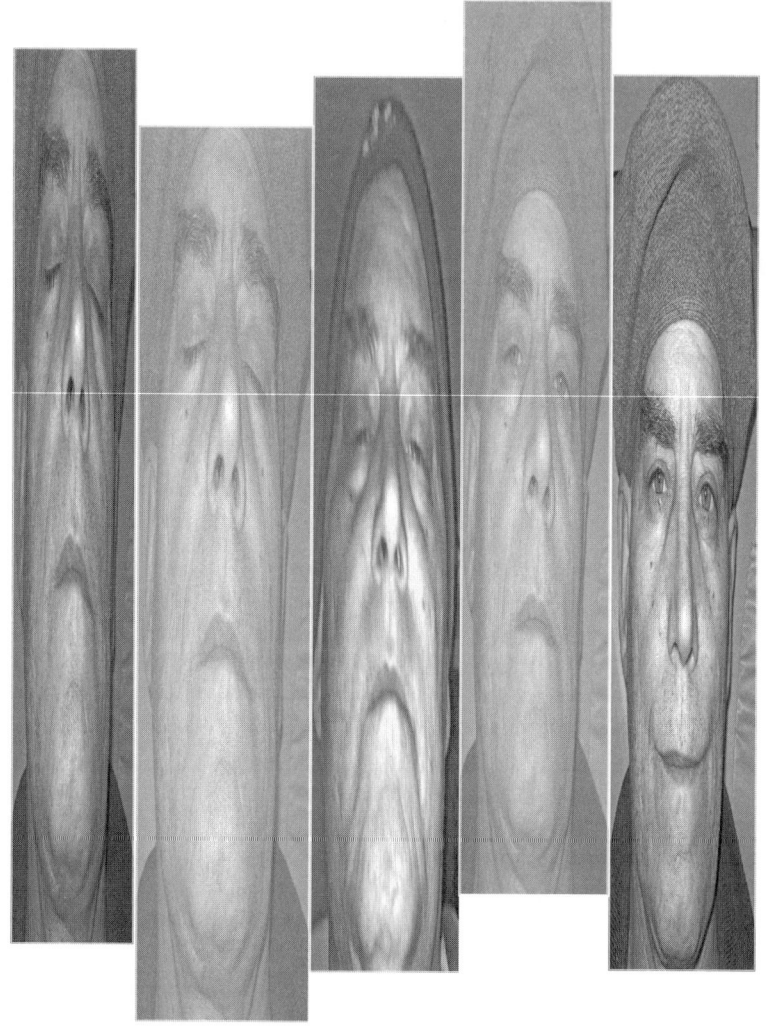

Chemo Brain *(Lame Medical Definition)*: a widely used term, it's misleading. It's not yet clear that chemotherapy is the mild cognitive impairment that causes concentration and memory problems in cancer survivors. Many cancer survivors with memory problems still score well on cognitive tests, leaving doctors wondering whether chemo brain really exists.*

---

*Of course Chemo Brain exists, look at me! I'm fried FrankenFred. I look like Jacob Marley in *A Christmas Carol*. Scrooge, I wear the chemo chain I forged in life. Boooooo!

CHEMO BRAIN

I'M ON A JET-LAGGED SPACEWALK CAUGHT IN A LOW-ECONOMY FLIGHT OF DARK ENERGY AND DEAD AIR. There's nothing I can do. Many of us are trapped in the sluggish weariness of the Chemo Galaxy. Lost in the present tense. We are time lapsed in space. There's no day or night. There is only the clinching weightlessness of hope. I have to drift through the shifting gravitational pull of side effects. They're my asteroids. I can't focus in the hangover depths. I'm space walking. My umbilical cable is no longer attached to my life. I can see my capsule. Its door is open but I can't get back inside to return to Earth. I clasp to the surface of a passing bystander. Catching my breath and watching the planets spin about the sun. What doesn't kill me, makes me *weaker*. Tumbling without direction. Hospital robes and wigs and knit caps of the lost forever float about me in crush depth. An updraft of stars lifts and exhales me. There is nothing to harvest in an asteroid field. All I can do is maintain my deflector shield to gain enough time to recover from the point-blank drenching radiating blasts taking out the meteor shower inside me. Launched in an empty odyssey of blackness with a becalmed vulnerability. Who needs the unforgiving invincible when you're lost in time and space? The stars don't twinkle out here — they sear. I see others like me getting sucked up in their private vacuum. Some are limp, coughing, slumped or sleeping. Everyone's spinning, looking at each other with hurt burnt-out eyes and drawn faces and crackling-kindling smiles. We don't scream because no one can hear us. There's no hunger as we spit out our tasteless consuming constellation. Some submit. Their souls in full retreat from their bodies. They burn up upon reentry in the Earth's atmosphere and circle down the drain of despair's wide yawn. I can't follow them. The loose comets of thought propel me through the blunt asteroids of doubt and the defoliant limbs of the dreamless helpless. I swing from comet tail to comet tail, trying to work my way back to the capsule and regain command, lightly touching the numbed finger tips of passing floaters amid the cosmic debris. I'm in suspended animation, caught in a process that overwhelms but doesn't erase me. Splattered in neutral. There is more and more nothingness pushing apart our zones. So we all coast without fuel, flipping and drifting, partially dethroned kings and queens of the universe under the rising dawn of a cure in a reversed twilight world. Chemo is a dark vacation with lost luggage. I'm in an unfamiliar terrain because everything I see I'm no longer part of — even my own body has veered somewhere else without me. I'm pinned down in a marinating chemo-centric crossfire. I spread my arms outward. I'm thawing out in the opposite direction. The sun is amazing. Its grazing heat gives me a tan and dries out my tears.

MY LIFE IS SHOT IN THE SOFT FOCUS OF CHEMOSCOPE. It's like a concrete mixer pulls up next to me and pours nuclear waste in an IV-flume down my throat then the crew sends me home. Chemo takes me with its firemen's carry into a fully involved blazing slush of me. For eight hours in my five-day stand, I'm intravenously irrigated with toxic chemicals in my veins. Chemo rampages like a lynch mob through my lawless body, completely possessed, drunk on a pharmaceutical cocktail, ravenously and indiscriminately ransacking, looting and pillaging healthy and malignant and benign cells. Chemo is unaffected by the moral consequences of slaughtering the innocent along with the guilty. In The World Court of Medicine chemo takes the stand and defends its amoral actions by claiming it was "only obeying orders" — the doctor's orders. But the collateral damage is all of me. This rabid anti-carcinogenocide has rearranged the wiring of my cranial electric grid. It's short-circuited my synapses and soldered power outages in me. I've blown a fuse. I'm stuck in a sinking mental funk where ideas swirl like spin art and form partial images of some significance, but before the picture develops into any form of clarity, it holds at blur. Its special effects steal away the present before I can taste it. I can't grasp or follow anything. Thoughts are little jellied fish I'm trying to scoop out of a stream of unconsciousness but they keep wiggling and slipping between my numbed fingers. I forget names I previously had no trouble recalling. I draw a blank on simple words to express myself. I'm building half of a mental suspension bridge to link me with the other half concurrently built on the opposite stretch of the outside world. Instead of meeting, both halves end parallel to each other in the middle of nowhere — my chemo-soaked attention span won't connect. My concentration is scattered in a skid. I try to do simple tasks then I stop, wondering why I began them — it's like licking stamps and sealing letters into envelopes then forgetting who they're addressed to. My splattered brain cells are a Jackson Pollack painting crawling off a canvas. If my mind is a building, chemo has picked it up like a doll house, shook it up and rolled it down Mount Everest. When it tumbles to a stop, I'm staggering within the demolishment to see what's left of my dwelling. There are no walls. I wander. Nothing is in its proper place. The TV is in the bathroom. The toilet is in the bedroom. The basement in the attic. The floors on the ceiling. None of the light switches work! And the cable is out. All I do is bluntly stumble and trip over objects. An autograph seeker unable to find his owner signature.

CHEMO IS LIKE I'M NAKED AND WALKING INTO A CAR WASH. Instead of brushes, there are needles drawing my blood. Instead of water and soap, I'm sprayed and swept by a pressure-washing toxic cloudburst. Then I'm blow dried with radiation from CT and PET scans. It's like getting off a wild amusement park ride that made me queasy, dizzy and just short of nauseous and the inside of my skull is gassed with sulfur. My eyes have a sticky itch, as if I'm walking into floating spider web strands. A perpetual indigestion combines heartburn and gas and feels like someone put a painful burp inside my stomach then folded it over several times and sealed it. The flat-fist velocity of a chemo burp lingers and slices a thin taut horizon across my chest like a stinging paper cut and plants its pointed edges into my armpits. And settles in. There's a metallic taste in my mouth, as if the fillings in my teeth are leaking. And it's all compounded by an out-of-tune back-up band of sharp pains and drifty mental drug shifts, a sore throat, muscle cramps, wooziness. Sleeping through the hurt lessens its effects. I'm cold almost all the time. If I feel a cool light breeze, it sears through me like a serrated sudden gust of below-zero weather. I'm willing to take the full-on burden of this heavy hit, angrily suffering inside the swirling globe of this constricting sphere as it settles and inflates me. Every four to six hours I take three different anti-nausea pills. And throughout the day, I relieve the burning sores in my mouth by gargling with a mixture of baking soda, salt and warm water, followed by a swish and swallow of a prescription wash. I stagger, trying to jab my feet forward. I blindly peer through a waxed-up haze, coughing. I've lost so much weight *even my feet are thinner* and easily slip out of my shoes.

Actually, when I think about it, I've become high maintenance: Chemo is the most expensive suffering money can buy.

THERE ARE SLIGHT PLUSES IN THE PURPLE HAZE OF CHEMO. Too bad they're useless because I'm so wiped out by the treatment I can't take advantage of them, but these side effects would be beneficial if I was healthy:

CHEMO PERKS:

1. It stops hair growth so I don't have to shave. No nose or ear hairs.

2. Diet suppressant so I lose weight.

3. My allergies are gone. Chemo dried out all the rapidly reproducing mucus in my thick head.

My compressed world is retracting. I get winded going up stairs. After eight steps, I have to stop and catch my breath. And we have *three* flights of steps from our house up to the road. Chemo is also dropping my white and blood cell counts. I'm supposed to avoid crowds because my immune system is weak. If I get sick, it postpones my chemotherapy treatment. I didn't want to give cancer any time off. Besides, I'm so fatigued, it's easy to not want to go anywhere.

In the meantime, chemo has grounded me:

CHEMO LIMITS ME TO THREE HANGS

1. Listlessly sit at the kitchen table by a space heater. Shivering, wearing a heavy hooded sweatshirt, thick knit cap, sweat pants. I watch DVDs.

2. Curl up in a fetal position under blankets with headphones and listen to music or books and stare off into space.

3. Wiped out in a lawn chair on the patio deck and mentally swerve and gaze at the sun through my closed lids.

Anyone seeing my chemo-funk would falsely conclude I was depressed. But *I'm strong inside*. Time is a quivering position on a compass. It's like driving across lower Wyoming or East Texas or the New Jersey Turnpike — you just want to get through it so you can get on with your life.

When I attempted to read, the words slid across the page and whited out on the margins. So instead, I watched DVDs. I got hooked on the *Inspector Morse* series. My parents were big on watching British detective mini-series shows. Mom continually commented on each new discovery during the show, trying to guess the killer, while my Dad would tell her to be quiet because she was making it impossible for him to follow the story. I imagined them sitting at the kitchen table with me, watching the show. In one scene, Endeavor Morse is engrossed in a book, researching an idea, and jotting down thoughts. I started crying because I couldn't do that. Reading and making notes was crucial for writing or doing show-prep for radio or stand-up. I went downstairs and longingly gazed at my books on the shelves. I ran my finger across the leather bindings. Emerson, Twain, London, Lincoln, West, Grant, Whitman, Chandler, Thoreau, Hemingway, Fitzgerald. I have the time but I can't re-read them. My world of books has been stripped from me. I need to be connected to a creative force. Cancer cannot create — its malignant sprawl can only multiply and divide. *That's Division not Unity.* I went online and impulsively purchased the complete short stories of Anton Chekhov. I felt the need to bond with him again. Chekhov, a Russian country doctor, who stayed low to the ground and encapsulated an original pulse of people. Chekhov nailed it. His words lived with warmth and humor. There are veins in his vowels. When this chemo fog burns off me, I pledged to use the break in the weather to go through the entire Chekhov collection. I wanted the unimpeded poetry of human contact. *Being alive.*

CHEMO'S PRESENCE OFTEN JOLTS ME AWAKE IN THE MIDDLE OF THE NIGHT. Laurie is asleep. It's 4 A.M. The morning mist from my Chemo brain clamps a shifting foggy wreath that compresses and steadily thumps around my head, chilling me. I put on headphones and listen to Miles Davis's *Bitches Brew* (Eerie music, but then again, the moment calls for it. So I get my ticket punched and go on the ride.). I'm stretched out on the rack of sleep and awakening. A weird image and feeling takes possession of me. A halo of a shifting circular formation of silver clouds opens into a curving hollow recess. Looking above myself, I felt a rush of energy drawing my chest upwards. It was an opening that said a life is awaiting. I remain humble. But I believe I'm destined to be released from my mezzanine of awkward limbos. Then Fred-5 appeared. I remembered Nash Park in Clifton, NJ. The park had a hill and a playground with a rusty junked World War II Curtiss P-40 Warhawk. We'd roll down the hill to get dizzy and disoriented. It seemed like a steep mountain, but was probably a slope. And here I was lying in bed, tumbling down the face of a parallel cliff. I gently squeezed my drainage bags. They were full. I was always worried if I was asleep, a bag might balloon and burst. I removed my headphones, got up and went into the bathroom to squeeze out my portable urine udders. When I walked by the mirror, I stopped and flatly assessed my "appearance-related side effects." I'm bald, gaunt, drawn and pale, weary from the lagging strain of catheters in my back. I'm listless, flagged, tilting. My heart suddenly seemed to be pumping in reverse. A whirling whooshed a flapping, fluttering dizziness through my head.

I blacked out.

When I woke, I was splayed on the tiled bathroom floor. A 10,000-foot fall from consciousness because of a failed parachute. My tubes guide wires had become trip wires. I should have been hurt. Nothing was broken. Had all my teeth. My bulging urine bags didn't pop. Catheters intact. I know what saved me: surfing. All those wipe outs. I instinctively reacted to take this fall. The surfing world I built beyond me is also my lifeguard. A stoke is looking out for me. Still, I cautiously rose to my knees, as if the floor would give way. I start tearing up. No getting around this — this is as real as it gets. Then I gasped a thought: Who saves the lifeguard if he's going under? Certainly not the ocean.

I'M BACK IN MY RECLINER. I pat the warm bulge ballooning beneath my pants legs. I carefully rise so the tubes embedded in my back won't snag on the chair's arms. I walk to the bathroom and pull along my Tower of Power that's stocked with hydration sacks and chemo flavorings — I look like some weird carnival street vendor. When no one is looking, I do a little spin with the pole, like it's my dance partner. A nurse catches my move and smirks. I shrug and enter the bathroom. I place a plastic container across the toilet. The nurses call the container a "hat." It's a flat plastic strip with a cup recessed in its center that has centimeter markings with numbers to help me determine how much I peed. Sometimes during this process I quietly whimper. I think of my parents. I'm glad they're not alive to see me reduced to this. Mom died from cancer. Dad killed from a surgery to remove cancer from his colon. Mom was a heavy smoker and you couldn't tell her anything. She angrily refused to change. After Mom was gone, Dad never got over it. Mom did everything for him — brought him dinners, cleaned, did laundry, mixed his drinks. He compensated for the loss by going out to restaurants every day, but most of those jaunts were an excuse to slam down three to four straight vodkas at each meal. He wouldn't break his routine. He also angrily refused to change. And when they discovered cancer in his colon area, I warned the doctor Dad was a heavy drinker. My understanding was alcoholics could be bleeders during surgery. The doctor dismissed my fears. *But Dad did bleed.* He got an infection. My parents won their arguments — they died. But they did their job: they gave me a great childhood, Christmas, Easter, birthdays, Thanksgiving, college. Beyond that, however they wanted to live out their lives or depart this world was their business. I didn't agree with it. I had to respect it. As I drained urine from the bags into the hat, I realized that their love combined and instilled a strength in me they didn't possess.

Fred-9 appeared and gave me another perspective. I twisted my ankle badly playing baseball. Dad carried me to a doctor's downtown office. I had my arms hooked on his neck and he had his arms beneath my legs. Pedestrians looked at us, nodded, passed and smiled. Admiration in their eyes. Dad. I remember being so safe in those cradled arms, so protected. The feeling of security never left me. I was raised within it my whole life. It was a platform that gave me confidence. I never felt alone. His armed presence was still carrying me through a world of smiling strangers and chemotherapy.

I took the pen tied to a clipboard placed on the bathroom shelf. I record the time and my urine flow on chart, then write beside my name: "Whiz Kid." I add next my flow numbers: "Record Pee!" I exit the bathroom door, totter slightly, and grab my Tower of Power to steady and regain my footing.

The longest journey begins with a backward step. It's a start.

ONCE AGAIN, I'M LOCKED-IN MY CHEMO CURL FETAL POSITION under a heap of covers on a warm afternoon day. I'm shivering, huddled under the blankets. Our cats surround me. Groucho is at my feet. Brooksie is alongside me. Bogie is on my head, purring so hard he sounds like a distant airplane. A sharp-edged sediment abrasively drifts deep gulping pains down through me. I'm trying to slip out of its grip. Cisplatin rings my brainpan. Short coughs come out of nowhere. I breathe in the dry humidity of chemo. *Chemo let me go. Let me go.* Every time I attempt to outrun and escape chemo's effects I get pulled back. It's like I've been captured by a cruel Chemo Giant, who's toying with me. I bolt for freedom. The Chemo Giant reaches out and drags me back. *Chemo let me go. Let me go.* He's squeezing me. I belch a hollow echo and taste a heated emptiness. A vapid chasm settles in my chest. Emptiness does not move. It edges out in one place. *Chemo let me go. Let me go.*

I make my escape by clicking my iPod and listening on headphones to *What A Feeling* by Irene Cara.

First when there's nothing
But a slow glowing dream

"I'm hurt, kitties. I'm in pain," I whimper, my face scrunching, tears rolling and stinging my lids. So much is pounding over me and beading up like mercury. I mmm-groan-gasp. "I'm in such pain, so much pain."

The drive for health's upbeat is overpowering. It's broiling, knotting, bulging and cresting a building flexibility to make me stronger. A gushing relentlessness burbles forth for a deeper glimpse of the life. Its swell is the undiscovered spring I've tapped. It surges and a geyser goes off and sprays the shit out of the grayness and mingles it with the light I never knew was inside me, sprinkling tears all over my upraised face. All I have left is the music in the heat of my heart. Its notes cushion me from the impending void.

Well I hear the music
Close my eyes there is rhythm

I sense the presence of a dance partner. It's the spirit in me that fights The Big C. It irrepressibly flares in my eyes. My pilot light of soul. Its ignition courses through me and stretches out a grateful smile and improvisational movements. I'm pulling my own strings to topple the Chemo Giant puppet master. I throw my blankets off. I grab Groucho. We dance across the kitchen floor as tears and anger flow back into me. Groucho squirms but nuzzles close and lets me lead. My smile becomes a clenched fist that's a kiss of death for cancer.

What a feelin
Bein's believing

"Thank you, I'm so blessed," I whisper.

Within my counter-clockwise revolving cold front, the force of life squeezes out another determined step forward. I cry in gratitude. *I'm here.*

"I'm so lucky, I'm so lucky." I clench my fists and weakly but firmly croak over and over to each throb of pain, "I *chose* this, I *chose* this, I *chose* this."

MY BARE BUTT CHEEKS SLIDE ON A CLEAN COLD SHEET OF BUTCHER PAPER ON THE EXAMINATION TABLE IN CLINIC E. I'm mentally mired in the middle of an endless chemo slough. A nurse is redressing the nephrostomy bandages in my back where the catheter wires are plugged and recharging my kidneys. I have this procedure done every two weeks to prevent infection. The nurse asks how I'm doing. While I'm shivering, I tell her about my digestion, aches and pains. She asks if I'm constipated. I flash to Fred-18 having breakfast, my grandmother, Nana, who started every morning with an unnecessary and unrequested graphic description of her pre-dawn bowel movements. A different kind of B&B: breakfast and bowel movements. I answered the nurse.

"Well it's pasty," I reply, then do an mmm-groan gasp. "I'm tired of being in pain." The nurse puts fresh bandages over the catheters. "They say chemo really depends on the individual. I analogic it, I don't believe it. I think doctors say that because they don't want people to know all they're in for is a solid wall of pain."

"Analogic?" she said, confused. "Oh! You mean *analyze.*"

"It's anal something."

"Chemo affects everyone differently. Some people are able to work at their jobs during chemo, others don't," the nurse quips, matter-of-factly.

"So they're sick of their job and sick *at* their job," I said, hoping for a laugh. "Chemo imitates life."

Nothing. The nurse's indifference is reinforced by her step-by-step functionality. Tough room.

I put on my shirt, slouch and sigh, "Chemo is kicking my ass."

"Yes, it does that to some people," she again says matter-of-factly. "Chemo affects everyone differently."

"I had the shakes for hours, I was like a junkie."

"Yes, it does that," she repeats matter-of-factly. "Affects everyone differently."

"I don't want to answer the phone. Talking to people makes me weaker. My mouth is filled with sores."

"We'll give you something for that. It'll numb your mouth."

"You mean you could have given me a preventative *before* this happened to me?"

"It's hard to anticipate each patient's side effects," she said, then bluntly vamped, "Chemo affects everyone differently."

"Yeah, I heard you the first time you said it."

OH, CHEMO AFFECTS EVERYONE DIFFERENTLY, REALLY? Duh. It's a lame excuse oncologists play in heavy rotation. I heard it constantly. Well, if the oncologist can make you jump through the hoops of additional tests and exams to cover their ass from potential malpractice suits, then why the hell can't they give you preventative drugs in advance to cover *your* ass from potential pain? Come on, I'm running up thousands of dollars on my tab and you can't put a little extra sugar in my coffee? Again, their standard reflexive response engraved in a die and stamped in metal is: "Chemo affects everyone differently."
But doesn't cancer also affect everyone differently? If the medical field has advanced through years of clinical trials to concoct specific chemo cocktails and enzymes to target and destroy tumor varietals, in conjunction, why can't they also create a preventative cocktail of medications with their diagnosis to alleviate the suffering patients experience before their body gets shredded by chemo's spraying shrapnel of side effects? I'm tired of oncologists and nurses refusing to testify against themselves by pleading guilty with an explanation the chemo-affects-everyone-differently defense. I'm stressed out like a straining tennis net stretched in the middle of a heated back-and-forth exchange between Pain and a Cure. I'm expected to be a good patient, but you're not allowed to ad-lib. A good patient is supposed to sit like a ventriloquist's dummy on the oncologist's lap and stick to the doctor's prescription scrips as well as script:

> **Oncologist:** You were unable to eat today. Spent hours curled under blankets, shivering, and your joints are aching. I see you have cankers lining your gums. Even your nose is running. And you're anemic. I might have given you some medication to prevent some of these side effects. I didn't. Do you know why?
>
> **Patient:** (*Oncologist throws his voice into you.*) Because chemo affects everyone differently. (*Suddenly the patient squirms and speaks in their own voice.*) Oh by the way, I've lost all respect for you and can't find a reason to pay you. Do you know why?
>
> **Oncologist:** (*Taken aback.*) No.
>
> **Patient:** Chemo affects everyone differently.
>
> **Oncologist:** Hey, you pay me whether you experience suffering, live with permanent side effects, or die. Didn't you read the small print on the consent form? You signed it. You *had* to. Anemia, bleeding, constipation, diarrhea, fatigue, mouth and throat changes. That's to be expected. We're also covered against war crimes. Our goal: prolonging our lifestyle — er, I meant, prolonging your life.
>
> **Patient:** At least I know there are some things chemo *doesn't* affect differently. (*Pause.*) Physician, chemo thyself.
>
> **Oncologist:** Actually, we prefer to call it pain management.

Yes, chemo affects people differently. I see these differently-affected people in the hospital's hallways, sitting aghast with weighted heads of quiet resignation, stunned and clutching onto a caregiver for support, wincing from a newly felt pang, and suffering from the natural shocks the lack of their health-care insurance is err to. I'm one of those differently-affected, slogging through a knee-high chemical slurry, moving one-second-hand in front of the other against the suction of the chemo time clock that has my brain set on vapor lock.

Instead of compassion in the world of pain, these impaired physicians evaluate computer readouts and scans and develop a protective professional callous between themselves and the patient's pulse. The self-contained doctors are swiftly rely on schedules and procedures and cite results and turn us into prescription dart boards. The oncologist's prescribed menu pad enables the physician to give his conscience a waiver on the collateral damage we suffer recovering from their treatment. As the hospitals and clinics run up their charges, their billing system doesn't address one error in the stacked deck of their imbalanced equation: the pain I take home. You know why? *Because you can't bill a patient for that.* On one side, oncologists deal with cancer, but never give equal time to the other side — that's *my side*, and that side is experiencing pain and needs to reduce that pain to gain an advantage. They reclassify pain as "side effects," as if those are sympathetic and acceptable answers. Why do doctors call them side effects? There's nothing *side* about them. If they're side effects why do they hit me head-on? Last I checked, *I'm the one* experiencing nausea, loss of balance, difficulty hearing, bleeding, canker sores, and flu-like symptoms and who knows what else? *I'm the one* who has catheters in his kidneys. *I'm the one* with urine bags strapped to his legs. *I'm the one* who going through chemo, losing my hair. Is nausea a side order like French fries?

Going through cancer is a learning process. You learn what the doctors *don't* know or understand. Sometimes the patient's ignorance is compounded by a doctor's inflammation of confidence in their abilities or ambition. When you're admitted to a hospital that has the latest advanced care you can benefit or suffer from it. And in a way, you're in third place. First there's the doctor who compiles research and writing papers to advance their career and progressional stature, then there's the student beneath them, and then, in third-place, there's the patient: us. That's why sometimes doctors give us the impression they can walk on water because they're stepping on our heads as we struggle in a sea of pain to stay afloat. Sometimes we have to pull them down to sea level so to remind the doctors our blood is also our treasure too.

They're wrong. Chemo doesn't affect people differently — it's *oncologists* who affect people differently.

I adopted a little plant and kept it near me so we could get healthy together. I need to know a world is growing outside me. I avoided criticism of shade and turned to the sunlight to give my hope an even tan.

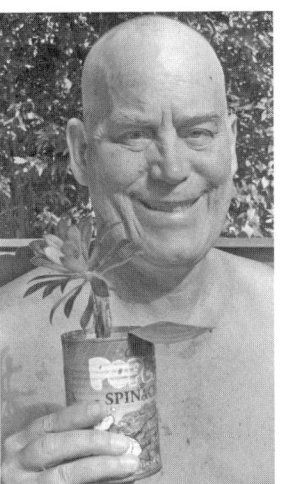

I STAND ON THE DECK TO WATER THE CACTUS IN THE POPEYE SPINACH CAN. The cactus has rebounded. The frail plant is struggling to grow in its can the same way I'm attempting to grow back inside my body. I smile. The cactus regained his strength to turn and face the sun. That's a good idea. We're still here, I think, this little cactus and me. We're good for each other. I gave this plant a personality. The same way my imagination gave me one. I thought of Fred-7 lining up one-inch tall, olive-green plastic army soldiers into battle on the living room rug, positioning them around furniture legs, and knocking them down by shooting rubber bands at them. After the battle I always left one soldier standing. Now, I'm playing with cactus in a can. I smiled like a child doing make believe again. And that's what the cactus and I were teaming up to make: *believe*.

THE SUN'S HEAT COOKS ME UP. I'm lying in a chair on the outside deck. The warmth. I'm giving off a low flame as if my body is a chemically-soaked log trying to burn off a layer of chemo white on my skin. My closed eyes look through pink lids as I drift in a toxic dead sea. I have heavy Polish bones I inherited from my mother. I can't float…except one time. After Fred-38 did a comedy gig in Ogden, Utah, on the way home, I stopped at the Great Salt Lake. Its waters contain brine shrimp and flies, algae, salt-water Kellies and Mormons. The saline water is dense. I slid in, laid back and instantly popped to the surface, completely stretched out, bobbing in the water. And on this deck, Fred-57 is floating again on my back in an indifferent Dead Sea. The air becomes a lukewarm liquid and soaks and saturates me and I break apart and don't resemble anything and everything goes soft, separates and hardens and I'm back, trying to stay afloat on breaths and hum a pleasant melody to a tune I never heard before.

My cellphone vibrates. I pick it up.

"Hello," I softly whisper, sounding like Babe Ruth giving his farewell address.

"Is this Frederick Reiss?" said an uninflected, hardened male voice. "You have a delinquent bill for the Stanford Hospital. Can we record this call?"

"No."

An uncontrollable rage rises within me. Billing me while I'm getting chemo. They call this health care? No this isn't *care*. I'm still sick! After all, I didn't run up these bills taking vacations or eating expensive meals at restaurants. I didn't live beyond my means, *my means is trying to live beyond me*. For the past couple months, I received bills for whatever my health insurance unfairly denied. This steady slew of invasive notices disturbed me. The late-payment fees were $35 to $45 a month. There was nothing I could do to pay these accumulating stacks of bills. So, I stopped opening the letters and put them in a file folder. After all, what's the worst that can happen to me? I already *have* cancer. Hell, they might as well cut to the chase and make it a $1,000 a month so I can declare bankruptcy quicker. Some politicians with excellent taxpayer-supported government medical coverage state everyone in the America already has health care because we "can always go to the emergency room." Last I checked, I don't think ER provides chemotherapy — unless every Wednesday a taco-wagon type truck pulls into the hospital parking lot and offers chemo, radiation, and vegetable wraps. Under our current health care system my body is on a reverse mortgage. Right now, my car has better insurance than me.

"Mr. Reiss, when can we expect payment?"

"Never."

"What?" he said, taken aback, which amused me.

"I lost my job. Months ago, I filled out all the financial assistance forms for Stanford. If I'm denied, I'll just declare bankruptcy. My insurance has paid a large percentage of the bills. Everybody's already made their nut. What I owe is gravy. I believe according to the law, if I tell you not to call me again, you can't."

"Hey, I'm just trying to do my job."

"I understand. You didn't want to be asking me to pay my bill anymore than I wanted to have cancer and talk to you."

"I'll make a note in your file not to call you."

The existence of health-insurance executives who enrich themselves by denying life-saving medical care to the sick are proof cancer has found a way to exist outside of the body and earn a paycheck. But one day, these metastasized for-profit professionals will become ill and lie in a hospital bed with an IV-needle in their arm. These over-educated, cost-cutting, bottom-line corporate ghouls might have excellent medical coverage without burdensome deductions or co-payments, but they won't be completely protected. The ghosts of all the people who died because their expensive procedures were denied by those empty pants suits and suits, those tortured souls will come a-haunting. And if you're one of those HMO shills and don't think blackened karma is closing in on your trail, I'll tell you this... I was *there*. I've heard the cries. I've *seen*. And you *will* be hunted and chilled by their last breaths. I can also say with absolute certainty, after all the chemo and suffering I've gone through, I wouldn't wish the pain I experienced on anyone — *even you*. But trust me, something far worse is coming your way and you can't outrun it because it's already growing inside you.

MY FISCAL RIGHTEOUS INDIGNATION GOES PROACTIVE. I throw down a call to the Stanford Hospital Financial Assistance Department.

"A collection agency called me," I said.

"Bills automatically go to collections, I'm sorry," a polite woman replied. "But it doesn't reflect on your credit rating."

"Yes, but they're still charging me penalty fees and interest. I sent a financial assistance request awhile ago."

"We're currently processing your application, if you get approved all those fees and the bill will be waived and taken care of by us."

"Well, okay, we'll just wait that out."

"If you'd like, I can request they don't call you again."

"I already told them that, thank you."

"Do you have anything else you'd like to say?"

"Yes, *I do have something to say*. You're Stanford Hospital. You have people who graduated from Stanford and good colleges but you are smart people doing dumb things. I'm going through chemo and you sic collections on me. It's stressful enough fighting this cancer and then you add even more stress to me by sending me these bills. Are you telling me if I get cured my life isn't worth living because I'll be in debt? Instead of caring you're acting like the Sopranos. You're kicking me when I'm down. It's immoral to treat people who are suffering this way. And you're listening to one of them. *I'm one of them.*"

There is a long silence.

"Thank you," she said. "I'll relay your concerns to others. We value feedback."

I guess this is yet *another* way chemo affects everyone differently too.

WHAT ABOUT THE PEOPLE IN MY LIFE WHO HAVE BEEN TO OUR HOUSE FOR PARTIES AND HOLIDAYS AND AREN'T HERE FOR ME NOW? They are the same people who never go to hospitals or funerals. Yet, they don't mind sharing and enjoying the *best* parts of our lives. But when you're ill, they withdraw. Then you see these people for what they *really are,* or *have chosen to be.* And if they're called on their shortcomings, they act like you forced them to try a food they didn't like. That's why they spit out their apologies instead of swallowing them. And they never forgive you. These same-old-shit-different-day people are always complaining about their job, spouse, or whining because someone else has more than them. They're never satisfied. They resent other people's happiness.

And they don't want to make your life easier because they can't stand their own lives. But I feel sorry for them, these people not only let me down, they failed themselves and decided to keep their life on hold in a world of self-reflecting mirrors or whatever limiting fear they use to restrain and justify their pathetic lives. They futilely circle the wagons to deny their own mortality — and by doing that, not acknowledge yours. How can they fear death when they're not alive? What they fear is *living* in this life. They console themselves by smugly and protectively squatting on their savings accounts and refuse to hatch generosity unless it's a tax-deductible charitable donation. They give themselves pardons and excuses they deny to others. These rule followers pride themselves on their ability to "pull their own weight." They use the personal sacrifices they made to achieve their own ambition as an example of the proper way to emulate a responsible life. But how can they call it a sacrifice if they're the only ones who reap the benefits? They are examples of people who fail to realize their bitter lives are *bad* examples. Actually, their lives aren't examples: they're specimens. They're a free fall stuck in reverse. Their globe gets smaller, grimmer with less daylight hours and becomes a hardened cyst laden with mushrooms in the darkness. They greedily cling to the wreckage of their broken life to anchor themselves afloat in a sunken past as the future drifts away from them. They're condemned to play a lifetime game of solitaire missing the winning card of compassion, yet they keep playing that game and losing and wonder why the cards don't turn up right for them. They refuse to expand the borders of their comfort zone beyond the circle of their limitations to include others. Their self-centered radius never overlaps or directly interlocks with people. Erasing the borderline of your comfort zone embraces you into a different world, a better one, a stronger one, and a happier one. Its interlocking and overlapping circle, and joins a more widening group of connected rings. Within each overlap is an improvised relationship you share with others that's filled with new recipes, party invites, unexpected gifts and experiences. These linked circles turn a chain into a necklace. It's the caliber of kindness. What people are capable of giving, compared to what they give defines them. Nothing else. So there's disappointment and joy on both sides of that heavily rubbed and worn coin of time we freely jingle in our pockets and debate whether to spend it on others or ourselves.

    The people who let me down have hurt me. But I can't judge them, because when you point your finger at someone, *three of your other fingers in the palm of your hand are pointing right back at you.* I can't hold their behavior against them. In the Book of Life we're all a little guilty of writing comments in the safety of the margins. I wondered how much I missed out on because I only highlighted and underlined the parts I liked.

CHEMO CHILLER THEATER

Creature From The Chemo Lagoon. Sometimes chemo turns you inside out. And you wonder, if chemo is the cure how bad is the disease? But with each hit you take, The Big C looks even worse. You have to become a monster to kill the beast within you. It's a fight, take a punch. It'll make you meaner.

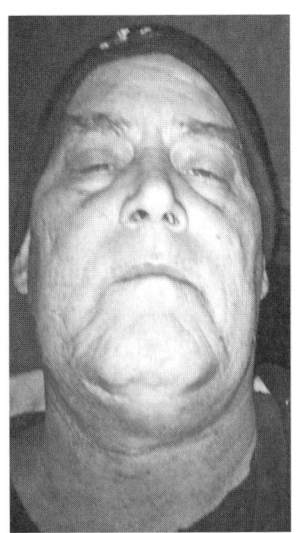

IN THE BLACK AND WHITE WORLD OF CANCER THE GRAY AREA IS CHEMO. The day is overcast — actually, everything is overcast. Most of the time I'm sleepwalking through my tour of duty in a muggy valley. I collapse into bed, trying to smother the nightmare of cancer. I do my chemo curl under blankets. I'm like an injured animal. Chemo's carpet bombing of pain binds me into a defensive fetal position. It's a 70 degree day. I'm freezing. I wrap myself in an electric blanket, as if I was attempting to cushion my fall.

Laurie arrives from work and finds me. I'm convulsively shivering. My teeth are chattering with each wave of pain that unwraps itself and rolls through me. She gets more blankets, places one after another on top of me. Tears line and flow over my cheeks. I'm saturated in pure toxic-laden seismic anguish.

It's like withdrawal symptoms from drugs or alcohol, only I'm experiencing the shakes in the reverse.

The drug's symptoms are withdrawing me.

How did I get here? I've been yanked from my stream of consciousness by an uplifting force outside of my world...

Dad and Fred-14 sitting in a rowboat, fishing and crabbing at Belmar Basin in South Jersey. Dad's drinking a Schaefer beer and I'm chomping on a ham sandwich with hot Kosciusko Polish spicy brown mustard on poppy seed roll and guzzling a cold Mountain Dew. We pull up the crab trap. A scrambling Blue Claw Crab is caught inside the water-dripping steel cage, jolted from his predatory crouch over the moss bunker head tied to the rusted wire grill. The crab is clearly shocked at how he was dropped from the top of the chart in the food chain of his ocean-floor world to the bottom of ours.

And here I am, crouched over the person I want to be again.

I blankly bleated to the emptiness, "I want my life back. I want my life back."

Laurie drapes herself over my blanketed body to increase my warmth.

Chemo's above-ground chilled trench warfare cloaks my flesh. My teeth chatter faster. My flesh is like jelly, loosely vibrating all over me. My stomach feels like it's made of dried-cracked mud that's draped over a wire hanger then winds around it in a stretch in a string of accelerating and building knots. A belch tastes like a foul methane gas. The burps become wet coughs that vibrate wringing aches throughout my lower body, then turn into dry heaves, loop around and begin again. I tremble under the piled blankets. I snivel short breaths that inflame the embers of the slicing, aching heartburn beating like a hostile pulse in my chest.

I slowly moan, "If chemo is the cure, I can't imagine how bad the disease is."

These tears, these warm tears, they keep coming. Cancer tears come with smiles. They come with hurts. They seek their own level and never seem to reach it. I wonder if this trail of tears is shaping me the same way water erosion creates a beautiful rock formation. The tears recede and leave a flood line of grief in bags under my eyes. I believe I will soon know everyone in the world. Because after emerging from this pain no one is a stranger to me anymore.

I *see* you.

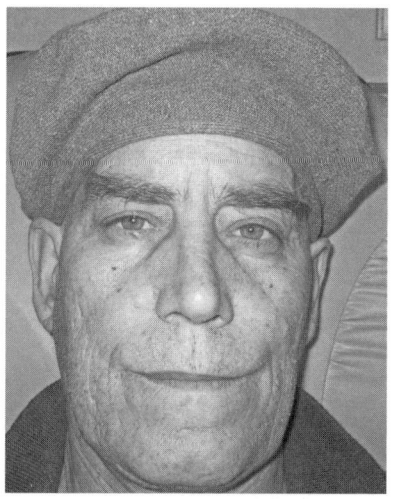

A Title Match at The Infusion Grand Arena
THE CHEMO KID
vs
THE BIG C
The Showdown of a Lifetime!

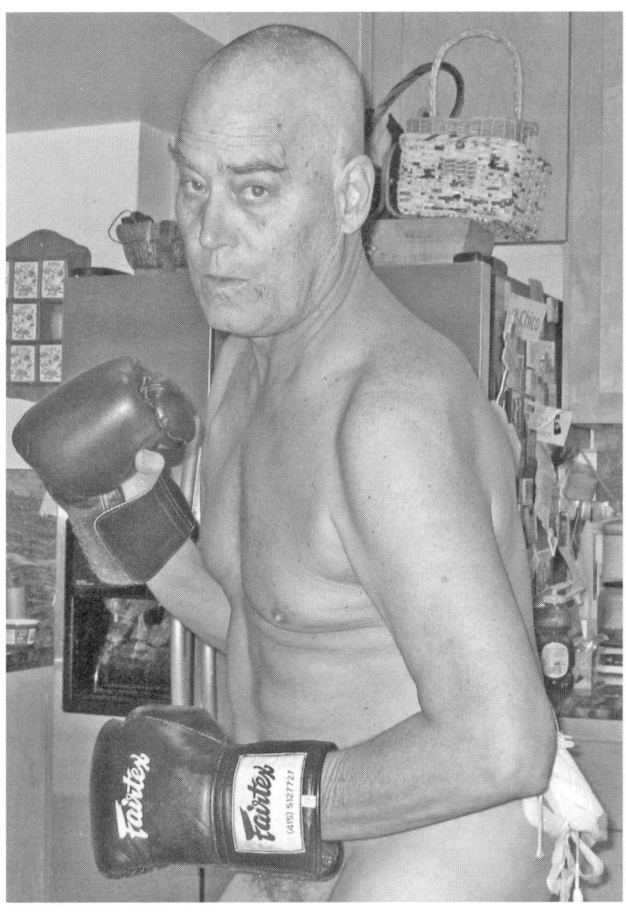

Round Two I'm in my corner, anemic and thinner. An oncology ring girl switches out the chemo on my Tower of Power. The boxing commentator says, "The Chemo Kid's vital signs are: Blood Pressure 142/93. Pulse: 76. Temperature: 97.2 Respiration 16. Weight 219 lb. 12.8 oz. The

Big C has clearly dominated this fight. In his corner, the challenger is throwing up He's a nervous wreck."

A bell clangs to start My Second Cycle of Chemo.

I'm flat-footed, wheeling along my Tower of Power. My gums are bleeding. I'm cold and shivering.

"The Chemo Kid's pins are already wobbling," declared the commentator. "Is he strong enough to handle The Big C's power? Early returns say no. He has everything going against him. A 57-year old man with a young man's disease. The Big C comes out swinging again. He's looking to put The Kid away. The champ sticks a stiff jab into The Kid. Right cross. Back to the left jab. Oh! Unbelievable! The Kid is taking shots to body, head, body, head. Punishing blows. Bing, bing, bing! The Big C's backing the challenger into the corner. The Chemo Kid looks done. He's got nowhere to go."

I'm like that zebra I saw caught in the lion's jaws, if I allow one more crunch I'm finished.

"The Big C is trying to end this. But his punches seem to be lacking the power he showed in the first round. Maybe he's trying too hard. He's wearing himself down throwing everything he's got. The champ has to be asking himself, 'What do I have to do to get rid of this guy?' The Big C tees up a right. Challenger slips around it. That missed blow left the champ open. Whoa, a short left inside from The Kid! That shot caught The Big C. He's hurt! Grabbing his side. He's hurt."

The bell clangs several times to end the second round.

I lower my gloves. The Big C has shrunk down to my height. I'm eye to whatever eye he has behind his soiled hood. The bulging muscles of his chest are twirling in tight silver spinning spasms. Gray lines dribble from his leaking tumor heart, like its mass is a dissolving pill in water. A glassy density smatters cloudy sections through his clear body.

"I'm not laying down for cancer," I hoarsely say, out of breath, clasping my Tower of Power with one glove. My free arm shoves the Big C. Tears streak down my face. My lips tremble and my voice quivers as I say, *"I'm growing inside you now,* you worthless piece of shit."

The Big C makes a move for me, then clutches his chest in pain.

I hold my ground.

He hesitates, then limps back to his corner.

"Ladies and gentlemen, we have a *fight*," exclaims the commentator. "Anyone who said this could be boring was wrong, and I'm one of them. This is more than a fight, this is a war!"

FOOD LEAVES THE TABLE BEFORE ME

THE NUTRITIONIST'S RECOMMENDED DIETARY WORLD BURNT UP ENTERING CHEMO'S ATMOSPHERE. Chemo grated my taste buds and blow torched my tongue into a pumice stone. Curtains of raw red sores adorn my gum line and upholster my mouth. When I was receiving chemo, volunteers came by with a cart and offered juices, water and crackers. Fruit juices scorched my raw-angry-red-cankered gums. When I swallowed water it felt like cut glass scraping my inflamed throat. Gulping made the back of my mouth feel like someone was rubbing sandpaper on an open cut. I grew to intensely despise graham crackers — it was like shoving cardboard strips in my mouth! My empty and dry stomach feels like a limp white piece of squid draped over a size-8 hook. I have no appetite because nothing had the right flavor. Almost all food tasted like dried leaves wrapped in tin foil. Everything unpleasantly became something else. Potato chips: wood. Popcorn: Styrofoam. Pasta: white glue paste. Bread: dry cotton. Meat: fur. Wine: a blend of crayons and lighter fluid. Beer: liquid sheet metal. Cheese: a slimy slug made of marshmallows. Coffee: lead. Cookies: hardened powder. Salads: mulch. French fries: sawdust twigs. Soda and junk food: chemical spills. Unsalted nuts: rotten wood. Cottage cheese: rubber cement. Bacon: oily pencil shavings. But I knew chemo hadn't permanently damaged my taste buds because broccoli, anchovies, hard-boiled eggs, cauliflower, asparagus, mushrooms and blue cheese *still* tasted horrible to me!

I'M CHAIN-LINKED BY CHEMO TO THE KITCHEN TABLE, hunched over in a chair, a blanket over my legs, and space heater beside me. I shiver and blankly stare at the rice and vegetables getting cold on the plate. I take one bite and push the dish away. I had no more appetite to shovel down this meal anymore than I had a craving for aquarium gravel. What I could taste determined my appetite. But taste is a temperamental vanishing act with AM and PMS. It's frustrating. Every day is different. I never knew what I'd be able to eat. Laurie scavenged for food in the shifting chemo wilds. Some days I'd devour fruit cocktails, cheese omelets, honey and peanut butter, yogurt, blueberry muffins, barbecued ribs slathered with sauce. Relieved I found food I could eat. But what was good one day, was terrible the next day, or even a few hours later. It's like breaking into an open field run and finding yourself without a goal line. Useless. Menus betrayed my hope's flavor. On a Tuesday, I loved carrot juice. Laurie purchased a gallon of it. On Wednesday, I spit it out. The gallon sat there for weeks until we poured it down the drain. We threw out a lot of food. Until I went through chemo, I never realized how much eating was part of my routine. Imagine waking up and knowing you can't look forward to breakfast, lunch, or dinner. Or an appealing snack to nibble throughout the day. I repeat, no snacks, no candy! No coffee! When you can't snack it prevents you from indulging your moods — chewing over your moods is a luxury of reflection between meals. And you don't have full meals either. It might sound unbelievable but I could go for days and hardly eat and not be hungry. When food tastes so horrible, it's not a thought anymore. Do you ever go outside and suddenly feel like eating pebbles, or separated remnants of truck-tire-treads or aluminum rain gutters? And wash it all down by lapping up a puddle of pre-mixed antifreeze in the parking lot? I developed a healthy distrust for meals. I knew how it would eventually taste like yard waste. Then again, chemo was ruining cancer's appetite, why shouldn't it spoil mine too?

THE PREMEDITATED NUTRITIONIST COMETH. I'm in a recliner, getting chemo and watching another season of *Breaking Bad* on an iPad. Walter White got mad at his wife and heaved a pizza on their home's roof. For a guy with cancer, he doesn't have many side effects, or lost his appetite. The show treats cancer like a skittish hex instead of a heavy-laden curse. I guess chemo lessens its effects when cancer is plot driven.

"How are we doing?" chirps the nutritionist, smiling.

Her skill-based support program is well-intentioned for her career, but a pathetic bureaucratic fairy tale to me. She looked good on paper. I didn't.

"You know," I politely replied. "I appreciate all your help and suggestions but just about everything you recommended is absolutely useless when you're going through chemo. Food hurts. Salads scrape my throat like paper cuts. Swallowing hurts. My mouth is so lined with sores that even when I tried to eat a banana its seeds ripped the skin in the roof of my mouth. When I brush my teeth my gums bleed for an hour or so."

The nutritionist sympathetically nods — she might feel my pain but *she doesn't have to taste it*. And she's clearly heard this response many times, and is able to deflect its poignant points with an upbeat message to justify her job. She prattles on, pushing her politically-correct yada-yada wholesome hard sell of drinking eight glasses of water and also maintaining a steady protein intake. She was giving me precise directions to get to a party I had no desire to go to. This was so pointless. She might as well suggest poison ivy instead of lettuce, razor blades in place of whole-wheat crackers, dust balls instead of frozen berries. Eat some granola but make a fruit parfait? With whose mouth? And, in whose world? When you're sick there is nothing more meaningless than well-meaning people with untested convictions trying to inspire you by constructive examples that they have never experienced and value judgments they never earned. Her intensity of belief was based in the comforting security of another world, a planet my body exiled me from, the transitory life form of healthy. The nutritionist kept yakking on. Perhaps, she feared that if she stopped talking, she'd disappear.

"I'll try," I said, wondering if I clocked her from behind with my IV-pole, would cannibalism be my solution to my diet? I say nothing else.

The nutritionist talks some more. I put her on mute. She decides to get scarce. She never visited me again. She realized she was suggesting a food diet to yet another one of the many patients who could no longer stomach her.

THREE RULES ON EATING FOOD DURING CHEMO FROM ONCOLOGY NURSES:

1. "They'll tell you to drink all this water and you won't be able to do it. They'll give you a list of foods that are good for you but you won't be able to eat them. The best way to get through chemo: whatever you feel like eating it's what you want. So eat it. You're eating so it doesn't matter what it is."

2. "If you know anyone who has marijuana. Get some. It helps food taste better."

3. "Don't try your favorite foods during chemo because they'll never taste what you want them to be and you'll never want to have them again."

RULE ONE: I FIND SOME GO-TO FOODS. My first great discovery... heavily buttered and slightly toasted salted bagels with most of the dough gutted out. I couldn't get enough of them. Why? *Because this food tasted exactly what it looked like: salted bagels!* I parked near Noah's Bagels on the Pacific Garden Mall in Santa Cruz, a block known for street performers and panhandlers. I was pale, gaunt, a bald tread of a skull under my floppy beret, wearing a hooded sweatshirt and shivering on a warm day. I looked like someone in rehab. I kept pulling up my sagging blue jeans from dropping below my hips. I dragged my feet past two disheveled bums, who were on a sidewalk bench in front of a cafe. They were drinking coffee and chatting. Cardboard signs with various pleas for cash written in black marker were at their dirty sandaled feet. But it was too early for the bums to squat in front of their signs and panhandle. They were starting their day with coffee *before they went off not to work!*

After I purchased a dozen bagels and walked to my car, no one paid attention to me. I didn't look *right*. I thought of when I fished for trout with live bait. If the minnow got hit by a trout and lived, and I cast the bait back out there, it was no longer the same vibrant fish. It wobbled. I was at one with those poor innocent trout-battered bait fish. Now, I felt guilty for piercing a hook through the thin silver tissue of the helpless wide-eyed minnow's soft puckering lips. I was defenseless. I could see why the elderly might carry handguns. If a mugger knocked me down, grabbed my bagels and stole my wallet, I wasn't strong enough to resist, and couldn't chase and catch him. No one wanted any part of me. Bums thought I was one of them and didn't hit me up for change, and pedestrians averted their gaze because they thought I'd ask for change.

Throughout my chemo endurance test, I didn't decide what was the best food for me: *it eats me*. Laurie found more go-to foods I sporadically ate at various intervals: oatmeal and brown sugar, tomato or spicy Mexican and Chinese soups, peanut butter, Wheaties soaked with milk until the flakes were soggy because crisp cereal ripped open the sores in my mouth. I'd sucked the moist flakes for one splinter of flavor. I was warned not to eat raw fish due to a weakened immune system. It had something to do with increased bacterial risk. But there were many days I had sushi doused with wasabi. Sometimes pizza worked. I'd rake my teeth across the slices, scrapping off the cheese and tomato and leave the stripped triangle bread pieces on the plate — the dough tasted like papier mâché, but oddly I liked eating the crusts. And liquids? I could no longer stand the Chocolate-malt flavored protein energy drinks. They went down my throat like thick paint. But I was able to down Carnation Instant Breakfasts, and cold Gatorade, and Arnold Palmer Lemonade Ice Tea. Laurie foraged edible snacks. Peanut-filled salted pretzels worked. So did vanilla caramels. But my most consistent go-to staple by far? Popsicles, Creamsicles, Fudgsicles, fruit pops. I'd watch a DVD movie or documentary and wolf down eight or ten in a sitting. The melting coolness soothed my throat, briefly deadened my sores. I loved being able to partially taste cherry, grape, banana, orange, root beer, pineapple, blue raspberry, chocolate, creamy vanilla. Wow! Why should I care if it was natural or artificially flavored? Salt is bad for me? Raw fish might give me an infection? Like I care. Hell, my simulated body is marinating and swimming in a dead sea of toxic chemicals! What's the difference? Who cares? *I can taste food*. What a glorious thing! When you're weighted down to the lowest point of your life, you desire any food that *tastes the way it looks*. And I've found some! I'm Sick. These Flavors remind me that I'm Alive, and give me The Power to Heal because it's making me Stronger. I don't care what it is, bring it! I'm eating what makes my chemo-ravaged mouth happy.

Taste is more important than substance.

RULE TWO: MARIJUANA DOES MAKE MEALS TASTE BETTER. I've been so deep-fried on chemo and meds, until the oncology nurses suggested dope might improve food's taste, it never occurred to me! That'll give you an idea the toll chemo takes on cognitive thinking. Really, how many Saturday nights did Fred-20 get stoned with guys at college and order pizza? A friend floated me numerous joints of medical marijuana. When I got baked, it enabled me to pan for flavor shards between the shrapnel metallic tinge of my chemo-altered taste buds. Dope had another huge bonus. Before bed, I'd smoke a joint and eat part of a hash fudge brownie or a marijuana-butter cookie. It helped me sleep through the useless hours and jittery minutes of my agitated chemo nights.

RULE THREE: WHEN YOU LOSE COMFORT FOOD, YOU LOSE COMFORT. During chemo I didn't attempt to eat my comfort foods. I couldn't risk losing the appetizing hope of comfort. *So I dreamed of comfort.* Turkey with mash potatoes and gravy — yummmmmm. Yes, Thanksgiving. Fred-7's plate had a huge mound of potatoes I arranged into a dam and filled it with brown gravy. An unsuspecting population of turkey slices congregated below the dam, unaware of the impending tragedy that will befall their quiet all-white community. I pressed the back of my spoon on the potatoes and breached the dam. Hot gravy flooded over the turkey-slice population. I imagined their futile little shrieks of agony. I swirled the potatoes and the gravy and the turkey slices into one gigantic light-brown glop, then salted and slopped it down. And what about a rare barbecued rib-eye? A greasy double cheeseburger with caramelized onions. Veal Parmesan. The crisp acidity of a chardonnay. Devil's food cake. Nachos covered with cheese and gleaming slices of jalapeños. A toasted tuna salad sandwich. Dipping homemade chocolate chips or frozen Girl Scout Mint cookies into a glass of milk. Taking a scoop of slightly melted ice cream that's hard and cold in the center but creamy on its outside edge? And fruit? The sweet curved white surface of a ripe honeydew melon slice. The pinching sting of a Granny Smith apple. And peaches! Oh, peaches! Biting and tearing the soft skin, gently striping away sweet pulp from a pitted scarlet seed and sticky nectar dribbling down my chin. *But memory was my most important meal.* When I was growing up in Freehold, those meals solidified the mortar in the building blocks of my personality. That's when pizza tasted better than ever. And Jersey beefsteak tomatoes, tremendous! Bread was fresher — oh, Fred-14 got up at seven in the morning on a Saturday and rode a bike across the highway to get hot poppy-seed rolls at the Shop Rite bakery. I can still feel the warmth of those rolls in the bag against my leg as I pedaled home. Oh, and what else? Chocolate-dipped soft vanilla ice cream cones from Jersey Freeze. Slices of Federici's pizza. Monmouth County Peanut Brittle. And Sorrento's submarine sandwiches — oh, biting into one of those oil-soaked hefty subs that sagged from its weight of layered meats. I'd love to have one of those subs now. But even if I did, I couldn't taste it. I wasn't thinking about death when I was eating those rolls, subs, ice cream cones, peanut brittle and pizza. The thought of that Fred made my lips purse together until my face scrunched and I was racked with sobs over food that was three thousand miles and fifty years away from me. The desire for future comfort foods in my past nourished a belief I'll taste again.

I can't eat, but I can feed the hunger.

URINE RACKING TIME! Everything I drank went straight to the urine-drainage bags on my legs. My creatinine utility belt weighed me down. I was bummed out about these bags. They restricted me from any activity. I couldn't even hit balls on a putting green, because when I bent down to pick up the ball from the cup and stood up, the Velcro straps loosened on my legs, and the bags slid to my ankles and the tubes tugged at the catheters and painfully pinched my back. I'd have to pull my pants down to adjust the straps. Who wants to carry urine luggage? I was elevating packing trash to an even higher level. Then I got an idea. I might as well have fun with whatever I'm stuck with. So I created *Lower Pelvic Cellars* wine labels and taped them on the urine bags. Looking back, I realize I should have called it *Yellow* Zinfandel. By the way, you know why they call White Zinfandel a blush wine? Because it's embarrassed to be in the bottle! Bada-bing, bada boom! One of my original vino jokes. I mean, I'm not doing stand-up anymore, so if I don't use it here, where else can I say it? The hospital tells me I'm filtering out my kidneys. I see my flush wine as a way to decant the cancer from my body. What do you do with a year that's a lousy harvest? You go with the flow.

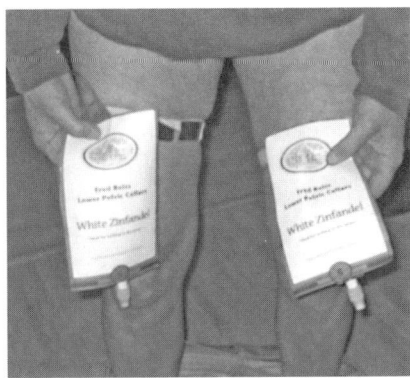
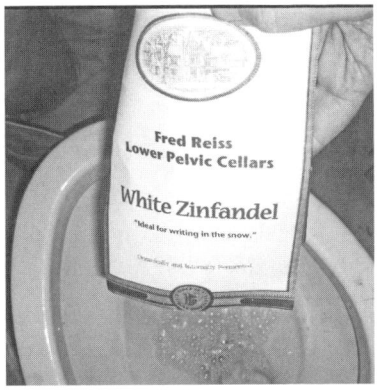

It's not a blush wine, more of a *flush* wine. It did give me an idea of another way to smuggle booze into a concert, theater or a long air flight. Who would want to check these bags?

FREDLY FIRE

AS THE WHITE NOISE OF CHEMO OVERDUBS MY THOUGHTS, I sit upright in the infusion staging area's recliner and mentally click through the 57 rosary beads of Freds, my chewable candies of sweet-sour mercy. I scour the shore of my past for some precious sea glass to reassemble my core. I'm attempting to find the connections and fuses and line up the holes with the screws so I don't lose any parts. In a way, I'm on an archeological dig, trying to dust off a delicate touch of a forgotten memory without shattering it so I can clearly define its shape, sharpen it, and mutate it in my favor against cancer.

I need to find living breaths without mortality. When I inhale, I imagine each breath is a year in my life and start at Fred-1. I think about my parents smiling and cradling me. I don't remember this, but I know they did it, and I feel that love. I randomly shuffle through my Fred beads. Inhale, exhale. Fred-8: Making contact with bat and ball in Little League and running furiously down the chalked baseline on my PF Flyer sneakers. The plastic batting helmet rattling loosely on my head. Wearing a baseball uniform with stirrup socks just like the pros, and I make it on base and for the first time *being in the game*. Inhale, exhale. Fred-15: He thought it was cool to go out in winter with wet hair because it formed a hard-webbed shell on his head. Inhale, exhale. Fred-32: meeting Laurie for the first time. Inhale, exhale. Fred-6: who cheered and pounded the sofa cushions as he watched Laurel and Hardy activate the wooden soldiers to save Toyland from Barnaby and the bogeymen in *March of The Wooden Soldiers* on TV. Yes, little Fred only believed in the victorious world of funny-men heroes! Inhale, exhale. Fred-37: getting genuine audience laughs when he truly locked into his style and firing on the stage, saying to a heckler, "You're proof you can have children through anal sex." Inhale,exhale. Fred-9: wearing a Monkey Division helmet, *Combat* trading cards in his pocket, heading off to play army. I'll need you to walk point! Some Fred Beads feel smooth and pleasant, others are like scuffed and burred. Inhale, exhale. Fred-13: In 8th grade there was an unattractive girl named Wanda. My buddy and I wrote her a love letter and signed some other guy's name. She believed it. We thought it was funny. It was cruel. The teacher exposed our joke to the class and chastised us for our behavior. We were jerks. We didn't regret our insensitive prank. Instead, we were indignant because we were singled out in class. I'm mortified by this bead of me. I'm no longer Fred-13. Yet that act cast one of Wanda-12's beads, and other schoolmates who haven't seen me since, might think that incident defines me. Was I also guilty of freeze-drying and categorizing others based on who they no longer were because of rejection or slights in the past? And told stories about what *others* had done to me and indignantly held their offenses against them, but expected everyone else to forgive and forget my behavior?

I look up at the chemo bag. It seems to drip the deeper pain of other people into me and drains away mine. I become insignificant. I don't mind, anymore. I have to leave the dead luggage of the past at the airport and take another flight. I seek the best sensations — when the vibrancy of an author's words hit me, when people liked me just for being me, when girls responded to me, and when I got a clue to aspire to be something outside myself. I stare at those ascending peaks before love ended, before dreams broke into skepticism, spurred on to plant my flag to stay where love remains.

I surveyed the Infusion Treatment Area. There was nothing distinctive about my clinical surroundings. Sterile doesn't develop a fertile soul. Whatever I make of my life is my best weapon against cancer. But there' isn't a trace of me in the Infusion area. I can't avoid my predicament but I can alter this environment.

My staging area needs a Fred makeover.

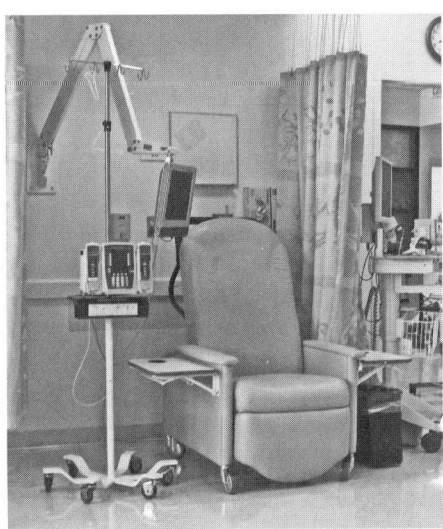

You can't change your situation, but you can improve your environment. I decided this place needed more Fred! Transform your infusion area into your world (*See page 94.*). Let cancer know you'll always be bigger than you are!

IF YOU CAN'T HIDE IT, DECORATE IT. On the next day of chemo, I placed a Beatles beach towel over the back of my recliner. At our best, when we become greater than the sum of all of our parts with someone else we become The Beatles, an energy bigger than we can ever be running on our own power. I fluff up an afghan blanket a friend lent me for butt support. And all around me, position framed photos from different periods of my life and between the Get-Well cards arranged my novels and insult book. I look at the photos and the cards and think of all the friends who volunteered to drive me and how Laurie was right there for me and how Maggie shaved my head and a week later brought me soups and protein drinks and how Linda Watson who owned DVD TO GO didn't charge me for any DVD rentals and Joey Greer come down our steps and took out our garbage and my surf buddies who helped me up and down the stairs to the beach and all these kindnesses coming at me and friends who brought me medicinal dope, hash brownies, marijuana-butter cookies and books and CDs. I got worked up. I started crying. Not for myself. I became upset when I reflected upon all the people who cared about me. I want to keep them — they're the life I made. Without them I don't have a life. I want more of them.

"You have all these pictures? This is so great. Who are all these people?" asked an oncology nurse, smiling at the gallery adorning my recliner. She pointed at the photo of a stocky man standing with a rifle by three dead deer. "Who is he?"

"That's my grandfather, Pop Pop, my Dad's father, who I never knew. He shot those deer. Dad wasn't a hunter. I'm not either. One time I killed a rabbit with a stick and I felt so bad about it I never killed a warm-blooded animal again. Pop Pop wanted to get me a pony. I'd be a different guy if I rode a horse as a kid."

"And this picture is cute."

"That's Little League with the Pluzato Tiles team in Clifton, New Jersey. Dad's the coach on the left."

"You're this one," confidently said the nurse, pointing at a ballplayer.

"No."

"This one?"

"No."

"This one?"

"No."

I place my finger on a skinny 10-year old Little Leaguer in the team's front row, sitting cross-legged with an extended open baseball glove in his lap.

"Yes," she said. "That really looks like you too."

"Right," I replied, laughing.

"And what are these others?"

"That's me surfing at Pleasure Point. That one is me performing at *Comedy Day* in San Francisco in front of thousands of people. That's me getting make-up for a national TV performance. That's Mom and Dad dancing — they've passed."

"Is that your wife?"

"Yes, that's Laurie and me in front of the wine train in Napa. We're into wine.

I**f** you can't H**ide** it...
D**ECORATE IT!**

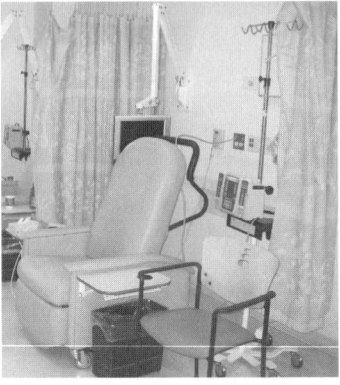

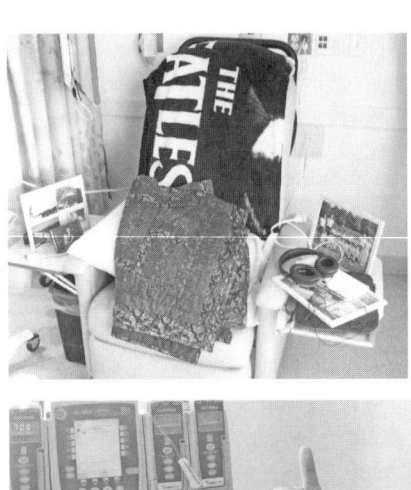

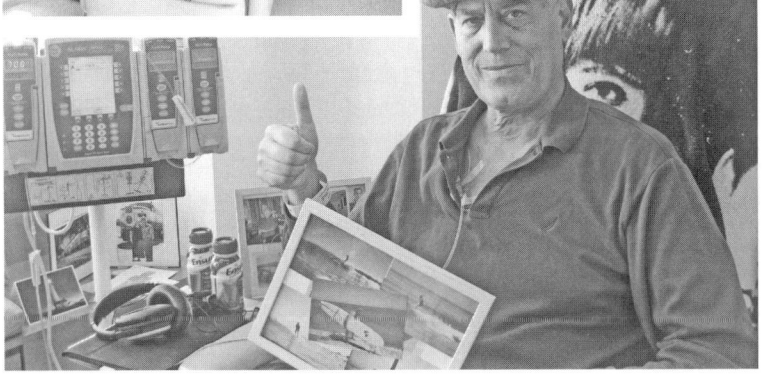

Your **LIFE** is yours best weapon to **FIGHT CANCER!**

To *SAVE* a life, *bring* your life!

So... ***BRING IT!***

Photos. Get-Well cards.

Music. Memories.

Anything that

Reminds you of ***YOU!***

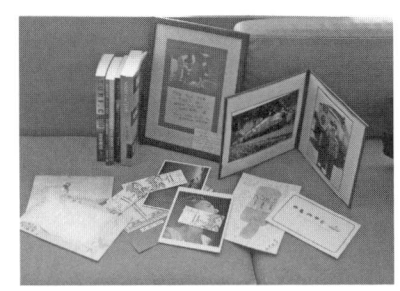

I've work at some wineries, helped out in crush, — even made some of my own wine: 'Fred's Red.' Named it after Dad. That one is me and my sisters and brother when we were kids — everyone was normal then. Today you'd never know the same parents raised us. That's my Nana, Dad's Mom. On Christmas, I'd get Nana from her assisted-living place and bring her to my parent's condo. When I went, I put a Santa hat on her and pushed her wheelchair real fast down the hallway. She told me to stop but I knew she wanted everyone there to see what her grandson was doing for her. I think I inherited discipline from her."

"You and who?" she asked, pointing to a different picture.

"That's me and Herb Alpert. When I was a kid, my parents always played Tijuana Brass records at parties. That music represented a great time. I had a chance to meet Herb and told him when Dad was dying and on morphine, I put headphones on Dad and played Herb's music so Dad would think he was leaving this world dancing with our Mom. Herb was a real gentleman."

"That's a great story."

"It's true. Oh, and that's me there, in a first-grade class photo. The only way my Mom could get me to dress nice for the picture was to allow me to wear my Elmo Topp's Lucky Cakes badge on my sweater. There's Mom in front of our old house in Freehold, NJ. That's where Mom was the happiest, and where we were happiest as a family. I went back there and scattered some of their ashes on the lawn of our old house. And said, 'You're home now.'"

"And what are the books?"

"Those are the surf novels I wrote. The other novel is about golf, and that one is an insult book I put together while I was doing stand-up." I paused. "This is the second time I've had cancer."

"Second time?"

"I thought I had enough depth after the first time. And here I am again, acquiring more depth. I could have done without it." I laugh. "All I can do is hold onto the things I love that fed and gave me strength."

"That's so nice," she said, admiring the pictures. "This is so nice to do this."

I shrugged and firmly said, "To save a life you have to *bring a life*, right?"

"That's true."

My words caught in my throat, tears started, and I warbled, "I have one."

THE SLOWLY COLLAPSING AND CRINKLING CLEAR PLASTIC POUCH OF CHEMO DRIP, DRIP, DRIPS. Each overdubbing drip accompanies the tick-tock beginning of *Image of A Girl*, a 1960 song by The Safaris on my headphones:

> *As I lie awake resting from the day*
> *I can hear the clock passing time away*

Chemo flows from the bag down the tube and into me. I flashed to how grape

When I was connected to the chemo-IV drip I imagined I was a vine trying to bear fruit. I needed the irrigation droplets so my pulp would be richer and larger than my skin's surface to prevent cancer from turning my heart into a bitter, sharp fruit. The vineyard was my support group.

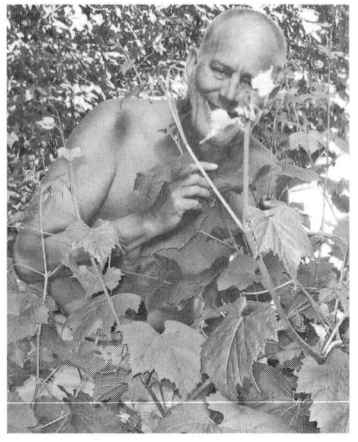

vines get drip irrigation in the vineyard. A vine can't stand on its own. The growing plant must be attached to a stake and threaded through a trellis. If a vine easily obtains all its water and nutrients, instead of driving down further for minerals to give its fruit more complexity, the unambitious roots settle for surface values and produce an out-of-balance bland fruit. A vine makes the best grapes when it struggles. Why? *It doesn't like to struggle.* Budding fruit is the vine's way of producing grapes for birds to eat and transport the fruit's seeds somewhere else. I'm in reverse growth. This chemo drip is driving my roots deeper into periods and memories, fusing my past into a future life. Slowly, neglected or faded moments acquire a jeweled clarity. But cancer is playing a deceptive game. My soul is rooted in the dark and well-drained rocky soil of struggle, but cancer is trying to sucker me into the upward pull of an artificial sun of looming salvation so I settle for shallow nutrients to feel sorry for myself. I drill deeper to my roots and outgrow myself below the surface. My drip stain of tears authenticates my refusal to form bitter fruit concealed under the wide leaves of green falsehood. Instead, my essence secretes bud breaks and burgeoning pulpy altered multi-colored fruit with acid and sugar and laden with seeds of sheer desire. Bring on the birds of freedom to take my seeds. I want out of here, big time! Fly me everywhere. Scatter me beyond this sick and twisted deceptive climate trying to weaken me to settle for less than who I'm worth.

"So, what kind of cancer do you have?" people inquired.

I flippantly answer, "The kind that can *kill* me."

One person dismissively made this observation about my dilemma, "Well, we all are going down the same road." I replied, "Yeah, and I'd like to call you a cab!"

Another phrase I detested — even when I was healthy, is: "This too shall pass." Just another well-worn platitude to conceal a person's indifference to the pain of others. I've always wanted to snap at them, "Yeah, this too will pass and so will you when I tell you to go fuck yourself." Give me a break. *This too shall pass.* Get out of my face. When you have cancer and stand at the intersection of Life and Death the only thing that passes is traffic trying to run you over.

Another observation: it's always the people without aches and pains who tell you to accept *your* aches and pains. The healthy blurt the most lethal comments.

When I got cancer people said, "Time to stop and smell the roses.'"

I'd reply, "A pig can smell roses. Don't take time to smell the roses, *plant* some."

Others shrug and pontificate, "When you're time's up, your time's up." Oh, they are so realistic about the deaths of others or their own death long before they face it. They all believe they're so safe and secure and accepting. But I bet, when their life is a second-hand click from meeting their mortal deadline, they'll frantically try call a time out or turn the clock back an hour so the alarm doesn't go off! They're hiding. They're also full of shit.

I BOTTOM OUT AND SURFACE WITH A CURE. I never saw it coming because everything started out worse than it became. It began at an appointment during the two-and-half week recess between my second and third cycle. I'm slated to receive a drug called Neulasta. I was kept waiting for two hours because administration hadn't verified if my insurance covered this new drug, an approval the hospital could easily have processed a week ago. Why did I need it? Chemo's multi-tasking goes after every rapidly reproducing element in my body, so along with cancer, it takes down saliva, stomach cells, hair follicles, as well as red and white blood cells. Red blood cells give you energy, when they're low I experience fatigue and need a blood transfusion. White blood cells protect me from infection. Mine are dangerously low. A Neulasta shot will boost my white-blood-cell count. What over-educated suit came up with a word like Neulasta! Sounds more like a diet drink or a tire-patching kit. The nurse said without insurance, the shot costs: $7,000! I bet in England or Canada it's 49 cents and you get a coupon for a free cappuccino. The shot is approved. I receive a simple "subcutaneous" injection (Subcutaneous means the layer between the skin and muscle, *which last I checked was still me.*), and like the pharmaceutical suits who inflated the drug's cost: the shot's a prick too. The needle is painless, but felt like the nurse was slowly squeezing a small wad of concrete into my veins. The nurse said the drug's side effects might resemble "flu-like symptoms and possible aches in my muscles and bones and joints." She wasn't even close.

A few hours after receiving Neulasta, I'm in my bed, wearing headphones, listening to Top 40 hits from the '60s. I'm clenching my blanket womb, tucked in my standard chemo curl, and shivering, riven with unceasing vibrating waves of pain crashing and splintering throughout my body. Neulasta is throttling my entire circulatory system. I thought white blood cells were the good guys protecting me. This is like being mugged by my bodyguards!

My teeth are chattering. I'm hugging myself. Slightly shifting my legs and hips to avoid getting entangled in my tubes. I'm flopping all over the place like a netted fish. I cringe in pain, wondering when this battle over my middle earth will release me. My eyes are passive slits. I get meaner. I want to thrash and rip out the tubes stuck in my back that are hooked like copper wires on the bolts of my kidneys. I crimp tighter to generate an internal ball of warmth to repulse the wind-chill of throbbing arctic aches whirling and clenching my bones and crimping my muscles. How long will this regenerating white-cell torture last? My reduced life is encased in a plunging pressurized submarine of silent and deep claustrophobic misery. Barrels of chemo and Neulasta depth charges quietly sink around me and detonate. The drugs' shock waves compress the delicate joints holding the hull of my riveted presence. I'm aching. Will I be crushed? My insides twist and bend back and forth. I coil tighter, trying to dive deeper to escape. Look at me. Half-filled urine bags strapped to my legs. Catheters in my back. I have cancer. I'm as low as I can go. Then unexpectantly, gutted and bottomed out on the ocean bed of my abdominal depths. *I hear the redemptive and exhilarating slapback percolating call of…A Cure!*

My organs are stirring and gurgling in my pelvic region. They're shifting, spreading, stretching out. *I feel it!* They have more room. Health is churning.

The tumor is *shrinking!*

I smile. Warm tears flow. I take several deep acoustic breaths. My stomach is growling. It hasn't growled for months! My chemo brain burbles out subtle meaningless fragile and gelid memories that rise to greet me. Here comes Fred-6, taking a bath in a blue tub. A dried-out green washcloth hangs stiff from the handle of the tiled wall's soap-dish rack. Fred-6 pulls the dried washcloth from its soap-dish perch and drags it through the bath water pretending the wiggling towel is a monster snaking in an ocean. Water changes the cloth's color to dark green. The creature is going to devour the plastic army soldiers on patrol along the tub's edge. The green monster slowly creeps up the blue porcelain slope, pounces upon the platoon and eats them alive within the towel's digestive folds. Fred-6's mother hears him screaming as he acts out the soldiers' deaths and the creature's growls. She shouts, "Freddy, what are you doing in there?"

Who knew who the hell I was then? Let alone what I was doing? On my iPod, the song *Concrete and Clay* by Unit 4+2 plays:

> *You to me*
> *Are sweet as roses in the morning*
> *You to me*
> *As soft as summer rain at dawn, in love we share*
> *That something rare*

I bend in bed amid the tubes, listening to the rumble in my abdomen as the green towel monster has returned to save me. It wraps around the tumor to digest its malignant indifference.

I'm winning. I'm *winning!*

Cancer's blood is in the water not mine. I've viciously surfaced into one aroused mean-ass, cold-blooded, lion-eating zebra! I'm laughing. The humbling tears of struggle gush out as I bind myself tighter as if my body is a human fist and sway to the beat of a tune I hear over this new horizon. I'm recovering and moving my feet and gospel singing a sixties oldie in the church of me that always believed in the invincible and inarticulate future I couldn't express inside me back then, but knew it was a potential force I always possessed...

The sidewalk in the street,
The concrete and the clay
Beneath my feet begins to crumble,
But love will never die,
Because we'll see the mountains tumble
Before we say goodbye...

The damp green monster is dehydrating cancer. The moistened green towel roars and I imagine the tumor screaming. I think, go green towel, go green towel! I'm laughing. Take this thing down, take it down!

That's the way
Mmm, that's the way it's meant to be

Green monster, I had forgotten you. Who can possibly know the true powers that lurk within a faded and latent washcloth?

TODAY'S GOAL: SHED THE CATHETERS AND TRASH THESE URINE BAGS BEFORE I START MY THIRD CYCLE OF CHEMO. I'm back planting my thinning buns on the cool butcher paper of the examination table in Clinic E. I'm looking at the woodenly beguiling barely lukewarm presence of Dr. Sri Lanka. Ms. Karma with a stethoscope. I view her the same way I see the tumor: an adversary to overcome by establishing and advocating my presence. Basically, I decided to maintain a professional distance from her to provide myself with the most effective treatment. Two can play this game, right?

"How much does a tumor shrink after each chemo treatment?" I asked.

She clips, "It averages to about 20 percent."

"So, I can get these bags removed before my third cycle of chemo?"

"No, you must continue with the bags through the entire treatment."

"After two treatments that's 40 percent. My ureters are free. Why can't these bags can be removed? My creatinine is down to 1.6 from 2.4. I *feel* the tumor getting smaller." I add with a slight urgency, "I'm urinating more through my penis instead of the bags. My organs are shifting. My stomach has never growled before. The swelling in my right foot is gone. I can't swim, run, or get stronger with tubes. I want these bags removed ASAP so I can better take this disease on."

A chafed Dr. Sri Lanka quickly pops off, "No, that's not correct. The tumor could be shrinking in a way that still blocks the ureters."

Wrong reply! Wrong, wrong, wrongo!

How hard would it have been for Dr. Sri Lanka to respond, "You know Fred, I understand it's difficult to have those bags, and if you weren't connected to them you would feel better about yourself and have more energy to get through this ordeal. So, before you start your third cycle, let's do another CT scan to if your ureters aren't blocked. If they aren't, we'll remove the bags"

But she didn't say that.

I was on my pelvic region's goal line. It was time to make an audible call: "I believe the tumor has shrunk 60 percent." I pause. "I *know* how I feel.

She flatly stares like she's tolerating me. Actually, she's heavily chapped. Dr. Sri Lanka *clearly doesn't like to be challenged.* I think she expects her patients to do exactly what she tells them. After all, I'm not an oncologist. I'm just a slab of meat that has chills and shakes in pain and pukes, what the hell do I know? But I'm not wearing handcuffs, and my care isn't in her sole custody. I was dripping with chemo leverage, and I was damn well going to use every ounce of it.

"I'm not keeping these bags on me for another two months, not if I don't have to!" I added with a little more intensity and bite. "I want a CT scan to see if the tumor has shrunk. I believe my ureters are free. If the scan shows they're still blocked, I'll wear the bags, but I don't think I need them anymore."

She blinks and stares at me and says, "I guess we can do that."

I raised my eyebrows and fired back, "Well, then I *guess* you will then."

From now on, when it comes to fighting my pain and getting stronger to beat cancer, I'm ordering an item that's not on her menu, I want a Fred Without Urine Bags To Go!

I imagined Dad behind Dr. Sri Lanka, giving me a fist pump of approval, beaming as he says, "That's telling her Fritzie. Don't let them do to you what they did to me."

I STRUT AWAY FROM CLINIC E CHARGED WITH A PUMPED-UP ADVANCE THROUGH THE JAGGED TERRAIN OF A PAINFUL WORLD, trailing fumes-of-mortality. I stumble and groan. But I'm on the offensive through a desert toward a further oasis, ignoring the stark landscape's hallucinations. Dreams on my shoulders drive off the circling vultures of doubt. As the chemo dust clears, the night and shadows of elsewhere snap at my heels. Head bowed, dragging tubes. I track cancer's trail. I see the tumor's hazy figure come into focus a couple hundred yards ahead, wounded. I'm taking two steps to its one. *I'm gaining ground.* Tears form. A tingling concentric glow bursts and radiates a mushroom cloud within my chest. And it's propelling me forward. The Big C senses my approach. The fallout of my soul is coming to finish it off.

Computed Tomography (CT or CAT SCAN) A CT scan works similar to an x-ray. The body casts a "shadow" on film when it is exposed to the x-ray, much like when you hold a flashlight up to your hand and cast a shadow on a wall. All of the tissue that the x-ray passes through overlap on the image, making it hard to isolate different elements. A CT scan works around this limitation by capturing one narrow slice of your body at a time. Inside the CT machine, the x-ray tube circles around the patient taking pictures as it rotates. These slices can be viewed two-dimensionally or added back together to create a 3-D image of a body structure.

A dye (contrast agent) may be injected into your bloodstream to enhance certain body tissues. The dye contains iodine, a substance that x-rays cannot pass through. It circulates through the blood stream and is absorbed in certain tissues, which then stand out on the scan. CT can be used to view arteries and veins. Contrast dye injected into the bloodstream helps the computer "see" the vessels. Since cancer seeks a blood supply, it can locate abnormal growths drawing blood from the organs. 3-D images are reconstructed so the cerebral vessels and accompanying pathology can be rotated and viewed from all angles.

I'M UNDERGOING A "CT SCAN FOR ATTENTUATION" TO DETERMINE IF CHEMO HAS REDUCED THE TUMOR. A radiologist nurse positions me on a pillow. She is in her mid twenties, engaging. She places my arms above my head.

I said, "I'm doing this scan so I won't have to wear urine bags on my legs. I hate accessorizing. If chemo is reducing the tumor, my ureters aren't blocked, so they can unplug the catheters." I pause. "Chemo is the only time a guy likes shrinkage."

No response.

Great, another tough room. To be fair, she is focused on setting up my scan.

I'm lying on the slab ready to be loaded through the cylindrical hole of yet another of the many machines that look like a an industrial front-loading dryer. Above my head is silver object that's a cross between a ray gun and a syringe that's attached to tubing plugged into an IV. It will inject an "uncomplicated intravenous administration" of iodine into the medical port above my collarbone.

"With the iodine you'll feel a warmth, you'll get a little dizzy, and there will be a sensation that makes you feel like your wetting your pants," said the nurse.

"At least I'll have something to look forward to," I replied. "I'll just keep my body straight at attenuation."

No response.

She goes into the CT-scan control room. A computerized voice inside the speaker within the tube said, "Hold your breath."

I'm slowly slid like a loaf of bread on a spatula into the opening. The machine hums and a thin circular revolving strip spins within the white cylinder. It sounds like a revving jet engine. A warmth glows and spreads inside my crotch, as if I was getting closer to a campfire. It fades. The spinning stops. I emerge.

The computerized voice says, "Breathe."

After the scan, the nurse detached me and said, "Did you feel like you were wetting your pants when the dye went in?"

"Yes, actually I'm disappointed I wasn't really urinating."

No response. Interesting what passes for focus these days.

"This is tough," I said. "Having these catheters in my back wears me down."

The technician replied, "I didn't realize how much people suffered until my cat had lymphoma, then I thought 'Oh my God!'"

"Yeah, I can see that," I said. "I once had to put down one of our cats. I felt terrible." I smiled. "This is a little different though."

Funny, I thought, she had flipped over, arranged and front-loaded an endless assembly line of cancer-ridden patients, but it took a cat to get through to her. Everyone is different — some *less* so.

I'M MULTIPLYING AND DIVIDING AND CANCER IS SUBTRACTING. My instincts were right. I get the results the next day:

> **Impression:** 1. Interval decreased size and FDG activity of hypermetabolic right pelvic mass is patient's known tumor.

Within a few days, I'm back in Clinic E's examination room. Dr. Sri Lanka enters. She is smiling so I don't recognize her right away. Her personality is pushing its one-dimensional envelope. She goes over the results of the CT scan.

"Your tumor has been significantly reduced," she said.

"By how much?" I ask.

"It shrunk by 60 percent."

I lanced a hardened and leveled look at her, lowered my voice and intently said, "Well, I guess I know *something*, don't I?"

"We can remove your tubes."

"Oh," I sighed, the word catching in my throat.

After Dr. Sri Lanka clops away on her hard shoes, nurses remove the catheters from my back. The yellowed tubes and plastic bags are tossed into the trash can. I never thought garbage could be so beautiful! I've shaken my harness. *This is proof I'm getting stronger than the cancer cells.* I was right. I slide my hands along my legs and my back. No tubes. No wires. No bags. Only smooth flesh!

I walk away from Clinic E. A redeeming rising column builds in my pelvic region and rolls from my stomach through my chest and splats into the roof of my skull and coats me with a vibrant energy. Sixty percent of reconstituted me is filling in all the cracks cancer put in my foundation. I'm lighter on my feet. I feel something else…the possibility of building up enough speed to cracking the silent barrier with the fulfilled booming of hope.

NAKED AND TUBELESS. I'm on the outside deck at home. My feet are unsteady. Laurie comes out and assists me up the three short steps as I climb into the Jacuzzi. For months, the tubes and bandages on my catheters prevented me from taking a warm shower or relieving my chemo chills in the jacuzzi. During tubular restraint, I bathed myself by patting a wet towel around my body. After all, I didn't have to shampoo my hair because I didn't have any!

"Ooohhhh," I sigh, sliding into the warmth. "Oooooooooh."

I remembered how Dad and I dropped Blue Claw crabs into a pot and watched their dark shells glow and turn a bright orange in the boiling water. A new Fred is being cooked. The heat caresses me. I catch my breath — a slightly deeper one.

"Ooohhhh," I moan, immersed in a soothing and warming jet-powered current that's swirling, embracing me, like I was swimming upstream to a source.

Warmth, I have warmth flushing away the chilliness that has settled in me, unwrapping the tense muscular knots where the catheters were coiled and plugged. The flowing is stroking my entire body and basting me like a creamy embryonic fluid. I roll and spin in this smooth liquid-fumed hug.

I happily sob and gulp, *"Oh, this feels sooooo good."*

Laurie is crying too.

I SETTLE DOWN INTO THE GROOVE OF A RECLINER FOR THE THIRD CYCLE OF MY CHEMO BEAUTY TREATMENT AND WEIGHT LOSS PROGRAM. I'm sapped. My body has struck a tumor reef. I'm staring at empty skies and a limitless flat percodantic dead sea of etoposide, Cisplatin, Zofran, Decadron, Mannitol. If opposites attract, chemo and cancer have a lot in common. They grind you down. Too bad we just can't return our body, take another one off the rack and walk away, huh? It always got me that a tiny insect can be flicked off the edge of a table, hit the floor, and survive a fall that was a thousand times the bug's height. Wouldn't it be great if a plane crashed and you saw all these people crawling unharmed out of the wreckage? I was the reverse. I was waiting for the wreckage to crawl out of me.

I need the Fred 1–57 Corps. and music to escape. I wearily mmm-groan-gasp and crank up Michael Franti & Spearhead's *Hey Hey Hey* on my iPod:

> *Hey, hey, hey*
> *No matter how life is today*
> *There's just one thing that I got to say*
> *I won't let another moment slip away*

My head nods to the beat. My feet move side to side. Cancer ran my life aground. I'm mired with IV tubes. But now, my partially submerged body detects less resistance. There's a slight flotation, not enough to surface and slip free, but I rock, shift and creak. The Big C is losing its grip.

> *You gotta live for the one that you love you know*
> *You gotta love for the life that you live you know*

I'm muscling up, regaining footing in the deep gravity of my heart. My chemo-anchored body is uplifted by a slight tidal shift — like a light breeze, but it's more like a layered wind with the smell of a summer shower splattering off hot asphalt mingling with the humidity and the smells freshly cut grass, roasting coffee and barbecued food. It's a call to a rising awakening.

> *And we will ride until the sun*
> *Goes to the place where it begun*
> *And we will live to laugh and cry another day*

Inhale, exhale. I'm Fred-17, lying in bed. It's the first day of summer without school. My parents are downstairs in the kitchen talking over a muffled newscast on the radio and my sisters and brother are fighting over the bathroom. The house is a living thing. A thin bed sheet covers me but I don't need it. I look out my open window and see green and blue through the white lace curtains that the warm and buoyant breeze has sucked flush against the screen, as if the day was trying to inhale me into its spell..

> *I hold on, I'm trying to hold on*
> *Hold on, hold on, hold on, hold on*

Inhale, exhale. Fred-57. I land back in the recliner my fall from the past cushioned by the pull of a familiar breeze from the first day of summer and there's no turning away from that dawn. Now, there's a blooming bud break stronger than me — like when I paddled hard for a wave then felt an boost of energy greater than my own, driving me forward, giving me the time to spring up, drop and crank my surfboard into the unzippering spiraling flow of a set wave. As sick and weak as I appear, I feel *better*. I'm entering another stage of a Stirring You in The Inside Me. Vibrant alarms are everywhere. A drumbeat that draws you out on the dance floor. Rising sap dripping off a pruned branch. The first cast of your fishing line slapping the mist-steaming water early in the morning. The fresh chirping of a bird as winter fades. I'm passing from a time zone where it was dark and it's getting lighter earlier and lasting longer.

The only reason dreams fail is we wake up too soon.

Give chemo a workout.
Cancer is going down for the count.
Chemo has a half life.
You have a *full* life.

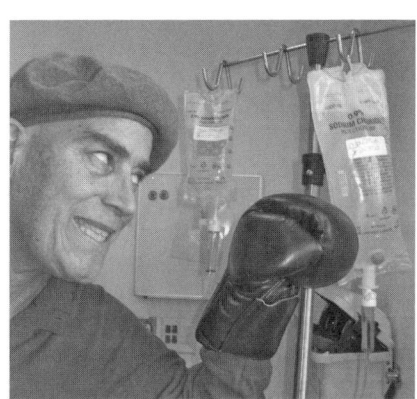

CHEMO SPEED BAG TIME. When I put on a pair of boxing gloves in the infusion area, I surprise the oncology nurse. It's March. My red blood cell count is low. I still get tired. My white blood cell count is through the roof. It's 16 times its normal level, something like 65 when the regular reading is 4. I won't have to get a Neulasta shot again, and that's good. I didn't want to know how long that "neu" would "lasta" again. The Big C's property value is 40 percent of its original assessment. I've increased my curb-appeal value by 60 percent. I outnumber it.

I brought the gloves to get me through this third cycle. At this chemo juncture, I wasn't too concerned about how I appeared to others. Why should I? Why should anyone? Ever.

"Would you please take a picture of me with these gloves on?" I asked the nurse, who was puzzled but impressed by my request.

She took a picture of me punching the chemo bag.

"That came out really good," she said, surprised and smiling at the picture in the camera's screen.

"Let's hope so."

She left. I put the camera and boxing gloves back in the gym bag. The gloves almost seemed like they were trying to punch their way through the bag's opening. I thought, this is where I am now, and this is what I'm doing to get through this. I have to be bigger than this place. Tears come. I worked the heels of my palms into my eyes, and smeared the warm tears over my face. They glistened, and soaked back into me.

Time to bench-press some chemo.

QUARTER PAST USUAL
SOME PEOPLE DON'T CHANGE

I'VE TRIMMED THROUGH THE CHEMO-CANCER SECTION AND STYLED BACK TO THE REFORMING WAVE OF MY SURF SPOT. My first day back surfing was the roughest. I was coughing and catching my breath, exhausted by the effort of simply getting into my wetsuit. I was bald and weak. I dropped thirty-five pounds. My wetsuit sagged loosely in places and abrasively rubbed my armpits. My limb are heavy, waterlogged with chemo. I almost fell carrying the board! I hadn't been out in the ocean for months, and that was months of sick, and still being sick, which is a lot different than being out of shape. But I was back Pleasure Point with a new board, getting a piece of me back, reaching out for the touch of day again. When I tried to catch a wave, my feet felt like they were shoe trees. I didn't have any flexibility to quickly spring up on the board to drop down into a pitching peak and surf. I crawled on the board. The wave broke. I was on my knees, stuck in the foam. The riderless wave peeled beyond me to shore. Cancer demoted me to a beginner's level. I was a chemo kook.

Over the next couple weeks, I couldn't surf but kept paddling out to rejoin the ocean's food chain. With each downstroke, I imagined I was climbing a liquid wall and said to cancer, "You're dying, I'm not dying!" Stroke. "Die, die, die!" Stroke. Stroke. Stroke. I'd cry and blurt, "You will not take me, you will not take me!" Then I stopped, pressed my lips into a clenched smile as warm tears rolled and streaked over my cheeks. My arms lost strength after twenty strokes. I pushed myself from a prone position and sat up on the board. My arms wobbled and my chest muscles ached, but I did it. This was my drill to get stronger. There's only one way to get surf muscles and that's in the ocean.

"Fred! That's you!" said Bill Farrington, a retired high school teacher in his sixties, who before teaching made a living for years commuting on a train to San Mateo to play the horses at the Bay Meadows racetrack. Bill went out of his way to track down my phone number and called me at home and offered his help. He was paddling in, but stopped, and said."New haircut, Fred."

"I'm getting chemo," I replied, pointing to my bald head ."A lot of people think I should keep this look. I'd get more waves because I look meaner in the water."

"Like you *needed* that."

I cracked up because I was known for zinging rude people with insults on the stage, radio and in the surf line-up.

"Yeah. I heard you've been coming out here every day. I haven't been surfing for years, but I *had* to see you just so I could burn you on a wave!"

I laughed and said, "No danger there. I can't stand up on my board, all I can do is paddle. You know when you surf and come out of the cold water and your hands are numb and your feet feel like they're made of marble? That's the way mine are almost all the time. I don't know what it is, but it has to be from the chemo. I'm not complaining. I know it sounds like I am. It's just something I have to deal with, wait out and hope I can heal." I paused, my voice cracked. "I'm just happy I made it through the section to the other side… so far."

"Well, I came here just *hoping* to see you," enthusiastically said Bill, who started paddling in. "I gotta go, I have to be somewhere. Just seeing you out here. It made my day!"

How can I not be touched, when I see how much me being alive means to the others around me? People can be so powerful.

I paddled in. Hal Stanger was in his street clothes, sitting on a rock. We surfed together for years. He called me every day. He had given me numerous rides to the hospital. He was smiling and said, "I was watching you."

"Man, I felt stupid out there," I said. "By the time I crawl up on the board, the wave is gone. I'm in the foam, and fall off my board like some kook."

"I was proud of you," said Hal. "You paddled all the way out there after all of what you went through. I'll help with your board up the steps."

After Hal drove away, I changed out of my wetsuit and looked at the ocean. Instead of being overjoyed to be back in the water, I was bummed and couldn't shake it. I stared at below-average surfers burning each other and gleefully catching waves — waves, I couldn't catch and once easily caught. I resentfully turned away to avoid seeing the fake-cool people surf and behave so badly.

Getting better doesn't mean a way of life hasn't died. My life is a jigsaw puzzle missing one piece. And I was that piece but couldn't snap back into the place of the world I loved. This gap settled an emptiness around me. Will I ever become that a missing piece? Or is my new life a puzzle I had to solve?

ANIMALS HEAR A DIFFERENT MUSIC. I once did a radio interview with a woman who rescued condemned abandoned pets from shelters. I said to her, "You never see a cat tapping their feet to the beat of a tune." And she replied, "True, but animals hear a *different* music." Then I thought, what about using a different music to crack the shelled claws of cancer's sprawling pincer movement? How can I compose a song I never heard? Well, we have three cats! Groucho, Bogie, and Brooksie. I had paws with claws in my arsenal to reduce the grip of this tone-deaf tick of a thing that has latched itself to sponge off the beat of my heart. Each stroke of affection from my hands to our cats is the only note I can hit to strum that different music. An affectionate pet is shaped by kindness. Cancer isn't tender. It gives nothing and takes what it doesn't have from your life. It doesn't lick you. It tastes you. Cats don't do that — if they have love. And it all came down to doing this:

> *Another pet for Groucho.*
> *Another pet for Bogie.*
> *Another pet for Brooksie.*

Groucho is the smartest and high-strung cat in our trio. Groucho doesn't meow, he squeaks like a rusty hinge. He's a stunted Maine Coon. Before we rescued him, he was an abandoned kitten brought to the shelter after being bitten by a dog. I taught him a trick. I put a treat on top of the kitchen counter and say, "Groucho, up!" And he leaps on the counter, then jumps away with the treat in his mouth like its prey. I briefly thought about getting a hoop and having him just through it for the treat. I decided that was a little to out there. Sometimes, if I'm sitting at the table, Groucho squeaks behind me, and jumps on my back. When he's between my shoulder blades. I shift and gently press him against the chair. He purrs, climbs around to my lap, crawls up my shirt and nuzzles his nose against my chin. I blow into his face and he sniffs. I cradle him in my arms, rock him, scratch his back and softly say, "Nobody hurts my Groucho." He purrs, places his paws on my chin, gently digging in his claws and looks directly into my eyes. "No doggie will ever hurt you again. Nobody hurts my Groucho."

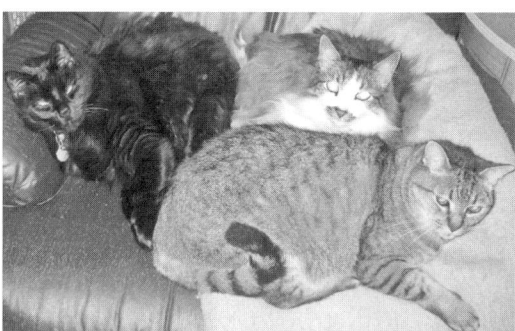

Each of my pets to our cats gives a kindness to animals who can't find it any other way. I think of all the animals in shelters and give our cats all the pets those homeless dogs and cats can't get. It's a sign language that translates to a larger affection for life, a desire for a life, a *value* for life, and generates and builds and infuses a rolling, healing and bridging force between us.

Another pet for Groucho.
Another pet for Bogie.
Another pet for Brooksie.

Bogie was taken from his mother very early. When I first held Bogie, he wrapped his furry black paws around my neck, purred, and nursed on my lactose-free ear lobe. A week after we adopted him, I picked Bogie up, held him against my neck, he didn't purr or suck on my ear. We took him to the vet. They treated him, but said Bogie had to spend the night in a clinic and there was a chance he might not make it. Early the next morning I checked on Bogie. I didn't want to see his green eyes fade from view. I took him out of his cage. Bogie's soft paws clasped my neck. He nursed on my ear lobe. I started crying and blurted, "He's purring, he's purring!" Then I whispered, "Bogie you got better. Bogie, you got better." The vet said, "I see a lot of cats, and you could put a leash on him and walk him like a dog. He's one of those." I replied, "I can't put a leash on Bogie, I just want him to be Bogie." Our Bogie kitten grew into a 25-pound mellow fur dude. And he's a picky eater! Laurie said Bogie is a Black Labrador in a cat suit. It's true. If Bogie hears someone coming to the house he growls. Bogie doesn't meow. He mea-yaps if he's lonely. Me-yaps to be picked up. Mea-yaps, plops down, and expects to be petted. Anytime Bogie spots a bag, he enjoys lying down and flattening it. His massive feline bulk has mashed its share of unattended bags of potato and nacho chips beyond recognition. If Bogie is resting and you say his name, he responds by slowly raising his tail, then resting it back down. Bogie. He's the biggest cat but he's the gentlest one who always concedes his resting or eating position to the other two. When I'm shivering from chemo in bed, Bogie sometimes jumps next to me, gently kneads his paws on my cheek, making muffins in my skin. He purrs and sucks my ear lobe. I cry and haltingly whimper, "Who's the biggest little guy? You are Bogie. Who got better Bogie? You got better Bogie. I'll get better. *We'll get better.*"

Another pet for Groucho.
Another pet for Bogie.
Another pet for Brooksie.

Brooksie was our first cat. He resented Bogie and Groucho. Sometimes Brooksie changes his attitude and licks them, then bites them. Brooksie is possessive for sure. If I'm lying down in bed he lays alongside me, stakes out his territory and hisses at Groucho and Bogie. If they ignore him and join me, Brooksie throws a snit fit and bolts. But whenever he gets an opening to have me to himself, Brooksie takes it. If I'm reading a book or a newspaper, Brooksie walks on it, lays down, and waits for me to pet him. When I come home, Brooksie runs up the stairs to greet me and follows me down to the house. Our neighbor saw this and said, "That cat loves you." In the morning when I get out of the shower, he comes in, gives my ankle a light bite, licks the water off my feet and looks up, searchingly. This glance means he expects pets. I scratch the spot above his tail and say, "Brooksie buddy, I know you love me. Brooksie, I know you love me."

Another pet for Groucho.
Another pet for Bogie.
Another pet for Brooksie.

The life-force of kindness pets. I stroke the living and the life within the cats transmits a different music that amplifies its decibels through my healthy tissue and crashes its rolling waves against the agitated tumor, acoustically eroding its malignant grip on my shoreline. My petting overwhelms cancer with ambient emotions cancer can't handle. It's wonderful to know love and tenderness can kill.

While I was getting infusion, I talked to a fellow chemosabi about the big C. He's a pretty moral and sensitive guy in his forties, a techie, who writes code on his laptop while he receives chemo for testicular cancer (It's his first at bat.). He's able to eat during his treatments. He's even *gaining* weight. I flipped him a few of my energy drinks. Most of the time, his wife is with him every day, works on her laptop, and goes out and brings him food. They purchased soup for me a couple times and refused to take my money. In the back of his mind, I'm certain he thought, things could be worse, I could be like Fred: he lost both testicles. But, I accept that.

"I haven't noticed any changes in me," he said.

I said, "Years ago, I got laid off and took computer classes to retrain my skills. There were quite a few of dysfunctional students who argued with the instructor on any reason to learn anything new. By the way they reacted to change, I could easily see why they lost their jobs in the first place. Then I thought, I'm in the same room with these guys so *I* must share something in common with them to end up here too. I faced it. I learned this: win your argument at work, lose your job. With cancer, all you can get out of this is: whatever you did before *maybe* brought you into this room — and change it. In a good way. Now, this is advice from a guy who has had cancer twice. So what do I know?"

"There is a tendency to slip into the same old habits," he said, concerned.

"No you won't," I replied. "You'll never be that kind of guy *because you said that*. When you catch yourself doing your usual routine, you'll instinctively pull back and resist it. You won't trust the guy you were ever again. You'll only go 80 percent of that way and stop. Then take that 20 percent and do something different. In that 20 percent you will find something else in your life that will change the other 80 percent. Trust me, you will never be the same. In a good way."

I wasn't preaching. This is one of the few times I really knew what I was talking about. We both knew what I said was true. Because once a truth is spoken, there's nothing to counter it but silence. I made him feel better. I felt like my life overlapped another person, and made a difference. In a good way.

I've been fortunate enough to be blessed with a new skill: I can help heal.

A DEHYDRATED AND BONEY GREEN GOBLIN CHEMO GRANDE DAME with angry body language radiating with resentful denial made a noisy and agitated entrance into infusion. I call her the Green Goblin because she has dyed green hair, a green blouse, short dress and shoes, as well as green-painted toenails and fingernails. She either left a St. Patrick's Day party, had prepared the themed outfit to attend one — or, there were side effects of chemo I was still unaware of. Her age was heavily tuned-up in her high-maintenance fifties but looked worse for wear from her share of way too much fun in the sun. Her skeleton looked like it was upholstered with the pocket of an old catcher's mitt. The loose flesh on the underside of her arms resembled beef jerky. Veins seemed to crack like blue tree roots through her skin. Gold and diamond jewelry adorned every limb and finger and probably weighed more than her. I wondered if she was half bombed, or aggravated because she was craving her next drink but could only slam down a non-alcoholic chemo cocktail. Nice people are quiet. Bad people are loud. She's *real* loud. She makes a big production to establish her presence. The Green Goblin flung her arms and stomped around a recliner near me. Her bracelets made a slithering chinging hiss. She fidgeted in the recliner and grumbled it was "impossible to get comfortable," then slammed down her purse, binder, and large appointment book on the chair's attached tiny tray. The Goblin's irritated nerve endings were loose electric cables, wriggling and snapping like snakes and giving unrequested shocks to anyone that dipped a testing toe into the shallow puddle of her being. She glanced over to me for sympathy. I decided to take cover behind my chemo game face.

The oncology nurse took the Goblin's vital signs, then struggled to insert the IV.

"You're hurting me," yelped the Green Goblin.

"I'm trying not to," said the nurse.

"Fuck you," snarled the Goblin.

After the nurse left, the Green Goblin consulted her notebook, huffed and snorted as she wrote checks. She treated the Infusion Area like it was her business office and everyone was her employee. My guess is she was pretty successful because she was clearly accustomed to getting her way. Except here. The Goblin only understood life if she was consuming it, now it was *consuming her*. She tried to act like nothing changed in her. It wasn't working.

She stopped writing, then sighed, "It's such a beautiful day. Everything was going so well. How could this be happening to me?"

I thought, how could this *not* be happening to you? I recalled when Mars, the male nurse, told me about the woman who went to see children suffering from cancer to feel better about her condition. I bet this whining sack of it's-all-about-me was *her*. Expressing sympathy for the vile Green Goblin was like feeling sorry for a shark that has heartburn after taking someone's arm off.

The Green Goblin's IV-pole's pumping machine started beeping.

She loudly decried, "Why is my machine making this noise? Where is my nurse? You can't just ignore me! You nurses do whatever else you want to do first, and then get back to me when you feel like it. I come here in the afternoon and you're still short-staffed and I have to wait. Why am I fucking here?"

My chemo dose was nearly finished for the day. An oncology nurse, a young friendly lady from the Philippines, came to unhook my port.

I said to my nurse, "If you want to take care of her, I can wait."

"No," she lowered her voice and said to me, "I don't go for that. There are a lot of sick patients here who are not like her. She should be grateful there are people here to take care of her." My nurse stood and shouted at the Green Goblin, "This is no good. There's no need for that language. You be quiet. You're disturbing other people. You be quiet. Here comes your nurse."

I whispered, "Ever try to find out why people are like that?"

She uncoupled me and replied, "It's a conversation you don't want to get into. They never accept where they are. If we don't come when they want something, they hit the emergency button. They don't think about anybody else. She's always alone. Whoever drops her off always has some excuse to leave right away."

The Goblin's oncology nurse, reprogrammed the IV-drip computer and stopped its beeping. But that wasn't enough.

She railed, "This is ridiculous, my pole is on the wrong side. The tray isn't high enough for me to do my work. It's on my legs."

When the nurse moved the IV-pole to the other side of the recliner, the tube connected to the chemo bags tightened and tugged the needle in the Goblin's arm. She lets out a disproportionate cry and flailed her jewelry-clanging arms.

"There's no need to be hysterical," said her nurse.

"Go to hell," snarled the Goblin, her legs kicking up the tray.

Instead of being rescued by her life, the monster The Green Goblin made of her life is coming to take her down. She is so caught up in herself she can't be hear the voices we all have within ourselves who are trying to save us.

Maybe the Green Goblin got the disease because cancer found its soul mate.

BACK HOME, MY MENTAL COCKPIT IS IN A CHEMO-CENTRIC TAILSPIN, I'm struggling with a joystick on the floor between my legs, frantically trying to pull out of a dive. I'm chemo curled in bed, wearing a sweatshirt and sweatpants, and a knit cap, under blankets, shivering within waves of pain, and listening to Rolf Harris's *Tie Me Kangaroo Down Sport* on the headphones. Fred-8 heard it on the radio my parents kept on top of the refrigerator.

"'Tan me hide when I'm dead, Fred,'" I weakly sang along with the tune. "Tan me.. I need heroes," I said to Fred-5. "Not Winnie the Pooh. I always thought he was stupid, except when he got his head caught in the honey jar — that stuck with me. And I got me mad that Eeyore the donkey never had a tail. Stupid. What else? I remember I listened over and over again to that Vaughn Meader album, *The First Family*, and tried to imitate the voices of the characters and do all the bits ("We must move ahead with vigor."…"The rubber swan is *mine*.") Probably I wanted to be a comic and didn't even know it, because I was one already. But, there was another role model…

Inhale. Exhale. Fred-5 lying on the living room rug in front of my parents' record player and listening over and over again to *David Wayne narrates Tubby The Tuba*. I got mad at the instruments in the orchestra who ridiculed Tubby because he didn't want to go ompah ompah all the time. I felt sad when the band mocked Tubby. He left and sat by a pond and felt all alone and misunderstood. A bull frog appeared and told Tubby no one listened to him croak his song out at the lily pads. The frog sang and Tubby played the melody. An inspired Tubby returned to the orchestra and performed the frog's song. The trombones stuck out their tongues, and the trumpets snickered. Tubby continued on and I cheered when all the instruments began to play Tubby's frog tune! And at the end, the frog appears and says to Tubby, "We have our points too."

"I forget Tubby's melody, but I remember running outside and down our front steps singing it, ready to take on the world," I said to Fred-5, smiling. "I think Tubby ruined us at an early age." Then Fred-9 popped in. "Oh yeah," I said weakly. "The DC and *Marvel* comics, and *Famous Monsters* magazines I'd spread out on the floor and trace the pictures in them. Remember when Superman was on that planet with the red sun and lost his powers. That issue spooked me. He was in pain and couldn't fly and his uniform got torn. How did Superman get out of that red-sun world? Oh right! He made it back to his Fortress of Solitude in the North Pole and reversed it somehow."

Yeah, heroes. Sometimes they are self-destruction enablers. Inhale, exhale. Fred-29, a reporter for the *Danbury News-Times* in the New Milford bureau office. After completing my radiation treatments, I returned to work and uncovered a story where First Selectman Clifford Chapin wrecked a town car late at night, and police covered it up. The next day, instead of standing by my front-page story, the editors badgered me, claiming they were getting complaints from town officials about my arrogance. I replied, "Seems odd, last week, you gave me an excellent job review, and complimented me on my ability to get along with news sources. I have the review in writing." The editor replied, "I couldn't find that review in your personnel file." I countered, "Well, it's a good thing I kept a copy." Then added, "You can say what you want about me, but all of these complaints are coming after my piece ran. I can write the article, *but you're the guys who ran it on the front page*." Most of the time, I think better when I'm talking, and after I spoke, I realized the local Powers That Be were putting pressure on advertisers, who then complained to our sales department. The result: it was either the editor or me who was going down for my news story. A few years back, an editor got fired because car dealers pulled their ads after the paper ran a picture of a car with lemons hanging over it parked by an irate customer in front of a dealership. Well, the editors had each other, I had no one but me. So, guess who was going down? After six years of experience, I was removed from New Milford and reassigned to an entry-level job in the boonies. Not all journalism is Woodward and Bernstein. The bad guys won. There's more truth in advertising. Now, I was covering Southbury, a small rural bedroom town where nothing happened, largely because its politics were completely dominated by Heritage Village, a retirement community of 2,500 condominiums. These seniors formed a voting block that rejected any tax, bond or expenditure. But on the plus side, my demotion propelled my resolve to leave for California. Actually, reporting on Southbury was easy because I didn't do any investigative reporting. I churned out bland features and articles. AIDS quilts at the library. Town Hall receptionists feeding ducks at a pond on their lunch hour (Accompanied by equally boring pictures I took for the piece.). New radar guns for the Police Department. How much sand the Public Works needed in its budget to handle snow on the roads. I didn't stop there. I churned out tedious and minutely detailed pieces on sewage assessments, siltation overflow in streams, zoning variance and education public hearings. Horrid stuff. It was kinda fun to be so boring. Being dull is easy! It comes effortlessly when you lack of ambition. I barely put in two hours a day, and spent the rest of my time, sleeping late, reading, working on jokes and doing stand-up on open-mike nights at the *Treehouse Comedy Club* in Norwalk, Connecticut, or sneaking off early on Friday to play in an adult softball league. During my reportorial exile, the editor who ran my the controversial story made an unannounced visit to the bureau office, telling me he sensed I was dissatisfied with my job. He was trying to provoke me into an argument to fire me. I didn't have enough money to go to California yet. I had to keep my job. I replied Southbury was a new challenge, a great opportunity to increase circulation for the newspaper. He left me alone after that.

Seven or so months later, I squirreled up enough cash, walked into the Danbury News-Times publisher's office and handed him my resignation, citing my unjust demotion. The publisher surprised me. He turned back my resignation and said he'd "look into doing something to resolve my dissatisfaction." I corrected him, "What will happen if I write a story about a politician who gets drunk and wrecks a town car? But I'm supposed to write about the little guys getting DUIs? If I can't go after both of them, I'm not going after any of them. If I have to pull my punches, I might as well be working public relations for Exxon saying how oil spills are good for salmon and seals. I should have been promoted for that New Milford piece." He countered by stating, "Fred, when Selectman Lou White attacked you months ago after the election, this paper supported you." I replied, "Yes, but he *lost* the election, if he won, I can't say I believe you would have supported me then. It's not about the job. This is a *moral* decision." Oddly, my conviction rattled him. We shook hands. I thanked him.

After I left the publisher's office, I looked at the reporters in the newsroom working on computers. Many covered their beats for five-plus years, and some probably pulled back from a piece that would burn their news sources and jeopardize their career. And oddly, isn't that what reporting uncovered, the truth other people ignored to keep their jobs? But journalists could do the same thing to keep their jobs but *hold others accountable* for the same moral shortcomings in print? Maybe that's why reporters are so cynical. There might be a future on another newspaper that wanted a guy like me, but I fell out of love with reporting. Like a cat that fails to squeeze into a drawer it once fit in as a kitten, I couldn't be that Fred again. I didn't fit. I couldn't go back. In California, I won unemployment because I proved the editors doctored my personnel files, so in a way, those editors provided start-up funding for my stand-up career.

Heroes don't always win. But my dreams dripped with sweat equity. My victory was keeping more of me, this gave me more star-power muscle to fight the red sun in chemo's world of hopeless yesterdays. Drifting between Tubby The Tuba, *Tie Me Kangaroo Down Sport*, and The Man of Steel, and struggling in my chemo curl for warmth within the blankets that formed my Fortress of Solitude, I might have lost most of my powers, but not my secret identity.

No oncologist visited me — or any other patient during the time I was deep-frying in chemo. They can say what they want. *But I was there.* All I saw were well-meaning volunteers wheeling carts and asking if we wanted water, apple or grape juice, saltines or those goddamn graham crackers.

I said to a nurse, "You know, my oncologist has never come to see me once up here. Funny, how you can take things like that personally isn't it?"

"It's the little things that count," she said.

I shook my head and said. "They aren't little things. They're *big* things because no one thinks of doing them."

A musician came into the Infusion Area and set up. Oh no, it was the glum woman playing that stupid harp. Great, Sylvia Plath with strings! Was she stalking me? She looked so miserable, which I found amusing. I didn't want to know her back-story, her front story was bad enough. She was human b-roll. I violated my comedy creed and made an obvious observation she had probably heard a million times. But I wanted to annoy and make her go away.

"I don't mind the harp as long as you don't have wings and a white robe," I said.

"Uh-huh," she snidely grunted, scowled and kept playing.

I wanted to pluck at the tube from my medical port leading to chemo bags on my Tower of Power and say to her, "You want to be bummed out, Harpo? Try doing a tune-up on this instrument for eight hours."

I FINISHED CHEMO FOR THE DAY. I sat in the hospital's main lobby and waited for my ride home. It's late in the afternoon. *All of Me* was coming from the piano, but no one was sitting at it. The instrument had a computer program that turned it into a player piano. The keys moved by themselves, as if a ghost in remission had returned to give us a concert. At least there was no sign of the marauding harpist. Then I saw a bald and pale child in a wheelchair being pushed along by his dad. The little boy was being treated for cancer. I turned away, hunched over and cried. When I was Fred-7, what was my biggest issue? Ripping apart pack after pack of wax paper-wrapped baseball cards, greedily cramming pink sugar-powdered sticks of gum from each pack into my mouth and thumbing through the cards and saying "Got'em. Don't got'em." And this poor child. This innocent. Dog-paddling in a whirlpool slurry of cancer and chemo. All his childhood knew was the pain I was feeling now. He was an old soul at seven-years old. Too old a soul for someone so young. How can anyone see a child like that and not feel we need to look out for each other more? It worked me up. Death hits me harder than ever. But pain to an innocent who fortunately has no concept of death? Years ago, a close friend of mine lost his son to leukemia. I did the eulogy for his boy because I experienced the loss of a brother to a crib death. My friend left the service, completely limp, as if his entire body hung on a wire clothes hanger. I mistakenly thought I shared my friend's loss back then, but today I truly felt all of his grief. I flashed to my brother, Matthew. He'd be 40 today. I'll never forget his small coffin. It was white and looked like a porcelain planter for flowers. Then I dialed back to a haunted and beautiful girl Fred-20 dated in college. A six-foot blonde with serious emotional issues I innocently thought I could resolve through kindness. If I met her in my thirties, I'd turn on one heel and flee any woman with that much baggage. But I was young. I believed people could be cured. I came of age in the 1970's — hell, I *came* everywhere! When I first met her she was wearing leather boots and trying to slide on the thin ice of the sidewalk outside her dorm but couldn't — that should have been an early warning sign. I grew up in a typical middle-class suburban neighborhood. She was raised by alcoholic parents in a Long Island beach resort community. When she was a little kid she had an uncle who had an erection as he bounced her on his lap and she went to an all-girl prep school and lost her virginity at thirteen beside her best friend to two of the school's custodians and as a teenager she masturbated with sausages and put them back in the fridge and watched her father eat them in the morning. One time, she came back all sweaty from riding a horse and we made love, afterwards she said, "I was trying to get you as dirty as me, but I couldn't. You're like a cork, no matter what, you just keep popping up." Her favorite song was *Miracles* by Jefferson Starship ("If only you believe, like I believe..."). In the summer, she had an apartment with roommates in Greenwich Village. One night we had the place to ourselves. After we made love, she left and went into another room, and without me realizing it, attempted suicide by taking an overdose of pills. She returned and laid down next to me in bed (Reflecting back on the scene, I didn't think I was that *bad* in the sack!). In the middle of the night I realized something was wrong with her breathing. She wasn't waking up. I tried to revive her. She threw up on me. She remained unconscious. I called an ambulance. When the EMTs arrived, one of them, a fat and ugly man leered at her nakedness. I sat in a chair by her hospital bed all night. She opened her eyes and said to me, "It's so embarrassing to wake up and everybody *knows*." I couldn't fill the credibility gap between her legs. Some people can only save themselves, and avoid confronting that responsibility by drowning their rescuers, and ungratefully turn on them, claiming they never needed any help. A few months later, she got an abortion — she was promiscuous so it might not have been mine, but once when we were thriving in the act, I peaked and heard the sound of a baby crying. It was probably mine. I never told my parents. One day, she calmly broke up with me. It took me awhile to find myself again. Beauty and sex have a way of making you become theirs instead of yours. I wondered if she had a relationship with me or I was an innocent piece on a game board she couldn't escape. Later she either found another playing piece or became one. She married some geeky financial guy, lives in Long Island and has a son. I knew her too well to ever want to see her again. Besides, I knew too much. But, I hope she made it to the brighter side. Still, she had to know in her heart she was alive because she was saved by a clueless boy who once loved what she could be — *and who she loved*. Maybe someone went away because of me, but one remained and reproduced another. I'd like to think I'm still in the plus column. But somewhere there's a minus with my name on it.

The kid with cancer was gone.

I checked the time on my cell phone: it was quarter past usual.

I PRESSURE DROPPED THROUGH THREE TRUCULENT CYCLES OF CHEMO STORM FRONTS. Today, the commanding cloud of chemo brain has cleared with a chance of slightly disconnecting showers. I take advantage of the break in the weather. I went to Pleasure Point. It was a sunny afternoon. The tide was high and swamped out the small swell, so only the fake-cool idiots and the desperate were in the water. I spotted two local surfers in their thirties. They were standing on the cliff. I never even knew their last names. And they didn't know mine either. Some surfers you only meet at the beach — you know, it's like people you only see at work, beyond what you share, they're not around. No big deal, that's how I was to them too. They had heard I was fighting cancer, but never called. I didn't expect much. Like I said, no big deal.

As I approached, they were intensely venting about the increasing numbers of rude people in the line-up who prevented them from enjoying surfing the waves. That's the way most surf spots go. They become popular. Soon there are so many ants on the sugar cube, you can no longer see the sugar cube, all you can see is the back of another ant. Today construction crews were running landscape loaders, hydraulic breakers, backhoes, and trucks, digging up East Cliff Drive, dumping gravel and repaving the one-way street that ran along the cliffs. They were laying out a future promenade and bike lanes. The two surfers glared at the work crews and bemoaned the landscaping improvements.

"The County put in seawalls to protect all the second homes of Silicon Valley trannies," grumbled one of the guys, wildly gesturing at the ocean, the road and the people. "And that's only going take the sand away and create more erosion. With no sand to buffer the rocks, waves are pounding harder into the cliffs. And the people in their nice $2.5 million houses are complaining about pictures and mirror shifting on their walls. On high tide there's a backwash warble on the waves that was never there before — it's going to ruin the break, I bet, just so these idiots can keep houses that they shouldn't have built here in the first place."

His middle-aged bro said, "Once this kook promenade is done, you know what'll bring? Even more goons, We'll be overrun by rude bicyclists who won't use the bike lane, joggers, people with dogs who looked the other way when their pets take a dump. It's the final coffin nail to the place, It'll bring people down here who aren't beach people. All I see are SUV people with SUPs —"

They spotted me and abruptly stopped whining. Whatever they complained about at the surf spot became insignificant in my presence. Nice to know chemo gave me clout and presence. They awkwardly uttered hellos.

"You look good," one surfer said.

"And check out the tan, you're darker than me," added his buddy.

"I'm trying to stay close to the sun, I lay out on our deck a lot," I replied. "I've been paddling out to get stronger. I can't really surf, I can't do it. So I've been coming here when it's flat."

"You're in pretty good shape."

"Lost a lot of weight but you look good."

The other guy added. "Yeah, surprising."

I pulled off my beret, rub my head and say, "I'm a skinhead now. I think I'll get a piercing, a tattoo, buy a skateboard and glare at everybody."

No response.

Tough ocean.

The rest of our talk felt forced. They glanced at me with goodbye-eyes not hello-eyes. They pitied me. I detested pity. I live in a no-sympathy zone: *Don't look at The Big C. Look at The Bigger Me.* What was I? A walking open casket? They pissed me off. I wanted to scream in their faces, "See my eyes. Look at them! Are these the eyes of a man who is going to die?"

Instead, I smiled and leadenly walked away. Depressed. In spite of my resolve, the two surfers carved out a hollow despair in me. Did they see something I didn't? I only had one more cycle of chemo left. Maybe I'm really dying and don't see it. Was I'm fooling myself? I couldn't hold it against them. I could barely handle holding it up against myself.

Am I in denial or is it just me?

A Title Match at The Infusion Grand Arena

THE CHEMO KID
vs
THE BIG C
The Showdown of a Lifetime

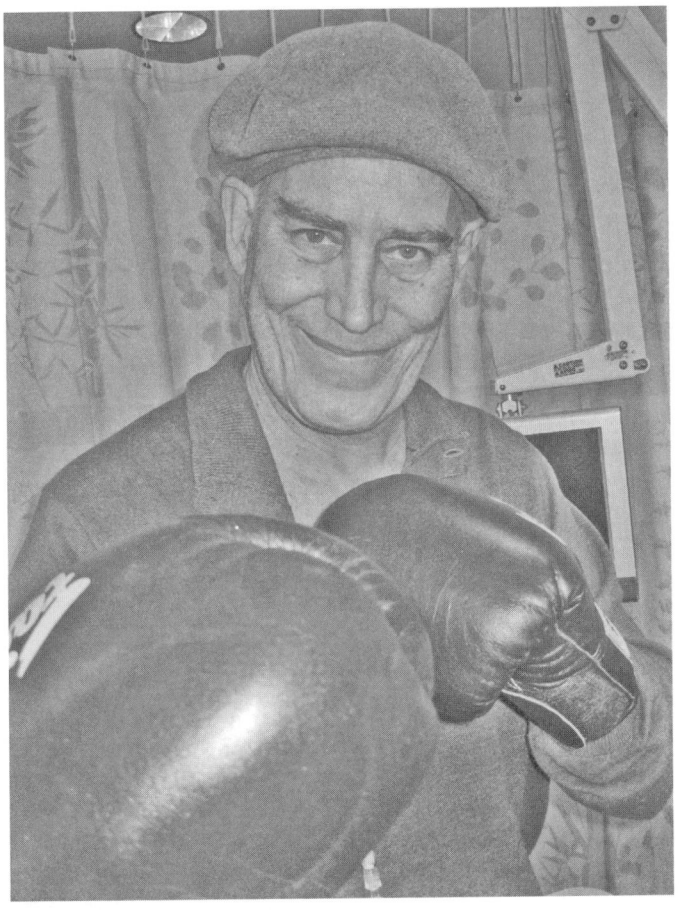

ROUND THREE I'M LOOSE. NO LONGER SADDLED WITH URINE BAGS OR WIRED BY CATHETERS. A newly arrived crowd fills the seats. The house lights reveal that the arena is filling up with all my Freds, and everyone else from each year of my life, along with caregivers, Chemosabis, and oncology nurses.

The ringside commentator says, "The Chemo Kid's vital signs: Blood Pressure 131/81. Pulse: 69. Temperature: 97. Respiration 18. Weight 210."

The bell clangs to start My Third Cycle of Chemo.

I stand on the legs of the IV-pole, propelling it forward on its casters by pushing one foot off the mat, like I'm riding a scooter to the center of the ring.

The ringside commentator continues, "The challenger is running on a full tank. He jumps from his Tower of Power and pastes a solid punch to the Big C's temple. Boom! That punch neutralized the champ. His feet are sliding."

My fist smacks The Big C's hood again. His head squishes like a mushy fruit. The Big C backpedals. I've taken away his chief advantage. He's a bully who can hit when you're not looking, but cancer doesn't have a clue on how to handle *being* attacked.

"What a left hook The Big C got caught with there! The Chemo Kid's bobbing and weaving, picking his spots," rapidly says the commentator. "The champ flashes a right. The Kid comes back with a left. Boom! They're trading hooks toe-to-toe. Pop, pop, pop! The Big C is staggering. Driven along the ropes. The Kid's got the champ in the corner. Unbelievable! The Chemo Kid is swinging wildly now: right, left, right, left! Hammering the champ. The fans are behind him!"

The crowd erupts in cheers.

"Another right to the champ's head," the commentator says. "A straight left jab to his mid-section."

"Suffer like I've suffered," I jubilantly hiss and heave another punch that draws thunderous roars from the crowd.

"In round one, The Big C was getting three shots to The Kid's none. Now, The Kid is getting three punches to The Big C's none. A right jab to The Big C's body. A straight right to the chin. Oh! A left hook to the head. Good night! The Kid closes in. The champ's against the ropes. The Kid is lighting him up. Upstairs, downstairs. I don't think the Champ knows where he is or wants to know because he's in serious trouble. It's critical mass. A right, a combination, and the bell sounds to end this third round and saves him!"

I lean into the The Big C. I smile. His clear skin cracks like thin ice and pulverized powder puffs out from his blistered flesh. His body is has lost its transparency. In his chest, the dark knotted tumor heart is blurred and streaming gray streaks. More and more crystals clot The Big C's liquid muscles, popping them like bubble wrap. He's deflating, shrinking within himself. Every spot where I landed a blow is steaming with depressions in the shape of my gloved fist. The brown hood on his head looks like a heavily dented can. His arms are wrapped on the ropes. He's rotting. Even his red gloves are losing their color. His insides are sloshing.

"You tried to take my life, now it's my turn to take you," I grunt to The Big C, smack my chest, and say, "You can run but you can't hide *in me.*"

TIGHTROPE WALKING ON CHEMO TO THE FINISHING LINE.

THIS IS THE FINAL DOSE IN MY FOURTH CYCLE OF INFUSION IS LIKE DRAGGING MYSELF OUT OF A CAVE-IN. You'd think it'd be my best day. But it's my worst one. Chemo dripped slower and slower than it ever did. It was tedious. I was jittery, impatient. Every unbearable second hung to me like a dangling syrupy chemo drop for a minute or so, then dripped to be replaced by another. Each passing minute made me more agitated. I still had 7 hours, 48 minutes and 3 seconds remaining. For months, I've been hacking my way through the cancer overgrowth and chemo undergrowth, chopping and scattering everything on a pile to be sorted out later. How long have I been beaten down while clinging to the star's cliff-edge of hope? The beams holding up my support system gave way under the suppressed stress and the accumulated enormity of my endurance test. The mental corridor that isolated me from life collapsed like a mineshaft. I'm buried up to my neck in empty test tubes from blood draws, discarded syringes and catheters, rubber gloves, used urine and chemo bags, empty pill bottles. How many times had I walked into a building that had "Stanford Cancer Center" on its doors? How many times can I be offered juice and saltines and fucking graham crackers? Taste sheet-metal tinged edges in food? Have a Huber needle snapped into me and watch nurses fill vials of blood? Record urine flows? Be lashed to a machine in a five-day stand for six-to-eight hours with tubes connected by a needle to a port implanted in my artery? It has a way of balding down your tread's grip. I crawl out powdered with chemicals, cough, and stagger away. It's a different kind of fatigue. I'm not tired on the inside. I'm weighted down from the outside, as if I'm wearing a burnoose made of lead. The steady drone of chemo settles coating after coating of a heavy dust on me. I can't brush it off. I'm a walking chemo layer cake. A ponderous weariness accumulates and numbs me. I'm incompletely in its elements. Chemo turbulence. My body felt heavier and heavier. The music on my headphones failed to take me anywhere else. I was stuck in this time slot. Inhale, exhale. My legion of Freds 1 – 57 were nowhere to be found. It was just Fred-57 in a recliner. I shivered and asked for warm blankets. I'm out of sync. My thermostat is broken.

I've developed an allergy to the dust of me. I was drained, tasteless, and burnt out. I had to lay down. I had nothing.

How can I lay down for cancer? I can't. I can't!

But then... I thought of Soupy Sales. Funny what you think about, huh? Soup had a kid's TV show on Channel Five in New York during the mid-sixties. Soupy created a warm world. His lion puppet Pookie sang and Soupy kissed him sometimes. White Fang and Black Tooth — all you saw were these giant furry arms with paws, and the dogs spoke in growls and grunts. The bad jokes followed by a pie thrown in his face. A guy who knocked at the door, and you only saw his arms and he'd often urgently plead, "Hey buddy, you got to help me!" There were so many of these grown men who hosted kid shows and injected bizarre comedy worlds in kids' heads. Guys like Chuck McCann on *Let's Have Fun*, who showed Flash Gordon serials and dramatically narrated the serial's beginning screen credits. Chuck did a great Oliver Hardy, and performed as characters in comics he read. John Zacherle who dressed as a Phantom of the Opera ghoul, kept his wife in a laundry basket, showed horror movies, and interrupted them by cutting back to himself in the studio, like during *The Mummy*, you'd see Zacherle wearing a pith helmet and peering around a column like he was in the temple scene, then back to the monster flick. I'd hear the camera crew laughing during their shows. There other kid show hosts, Sandy Becker with his Hambone and Norton Nork characters. Officer Joe Bolton showing Three Stooges films, Uncle Fred Scott, Beachcomber Bill, Captain Jack McCarthy. I went online with my iPad and watched old clips of their shows on *YouTube* to refresh the worlds they put into me. Their significance is a trivia question now. But what of the others who awakened me to expand my borders into something better, bigger, wider, happier? We all have them. For me it was Mickey Mantle, Laurel and Hardy, W.C. Fields, Humphrey Bogart, Mort Sahl. Don Rickles, Lenny Bruce, Groucho Marx, Abbott and Costello, Lincoln and Grant, Sleepy Labeef, Tubby The Tuba, Dean Martin, John F Kennedy, classic TV sixties shows, The Beatles, JD Salinger, Kerouac, Jean Shepherd or Don Imus, rock music, Herb Alpert, Bruce Springsteen, Woodward and Bernstein, or favorite movies I'd see over and over, or books I'd reread, and the so many others who multiplied and divided me to tilt my sensations to their calling. But now I was so tired. I was beaten, jobless, bottomed out on a cure. My dreams had nowhere to go. *I couldn't get through this last day unless I broke my vow and laid down for cancer.* I failed! Then pelvic region thrummed and radiated circular waves whose swell lines lapped out a pulsating tingling hum and vibration that lined the peripheral shoreline of my body. What created my dreams came to save me. Their magnitude wrapped a protective barrier around me, like an electrified fence. Cancer, to kill me, you first have to pass through all the heroes and lives and loves and take down everything that inspired me, and by the time you get to me, you'll be mine! My impractical heroes and irresponsible dreams tucked me in, I smiled and safely closed my eyes.

LATER I WAS AWAKENED BY THE CHIRPING CANNED MUSIC OF THE NUTRITIONIST, who was warbling her eat-healthy set list to a middle-aged man. He sat across from me. It was his first day of chemo. The nutritionist florescently flashed her whole-wheat smiles and yogurt-white teeth, unfolded the useless menu map of literature in her lap, and yammered through her well-worn freshman orientation on the importance of protein, hydrating yourself with eight 8-ounce glasses of water to flush out chemo, and eating small portions throughout the day.

When my half closed eyes glimpsed her new clueless pupil, I felt like a seasoned combat veteran who had completed his tour of duty and was seeing a fresh recruit rotated into my old unit who was replacing me. The gullible Chemosabi was cheerfully obedient, and overweight. The majority of newly arrived Chemosabis were amazingly out of shape. They didn't bring anything to the game. Their bodies said, "I get home from work, too tired to do anything but have a drink, sit on my butt, light up a cigarette and watch TV for the rest of the night." Their first infusion-plate appearance usually didn't tolerate chemo well — they went down hard, called out on strikes without swinging.

After the nutritionist left her prey, I went over to the new recruit's recliner.

"Excuse me," I said.

The Chemosabi looked at my thinned frame, sagging pants, and my bald head beneath by beret. His face had a cheerful uncomprehending acceptance of the unknown. The poor bastard. I wanted to help him. He had a needle in his arm. He didn't have a port.

"I know she talked about all the food you can eat, and I hope you can do it. But once chemo takes hold you can't eat any of it. My advice is eat what you like in the first week because you won't be able to taste anything later. What worked for me best were popsicles, Carnation Instant Breakfasts, and salted bagels. Don't stock up on too many things. What you'll like one day, you won't be able to stand the next day. Whatever you feel like eating, is the only thing you'll eat. It's almost like how a pregnant woman wants pickles or chocolate at midnight. You'll get sores in your mouth, ask the oncologist for a rinse and a numbing gel so you might be able to head some of it off before it happens."

"That's very good advice," he nervously said. He didn't want to believe me. He nodded. "I appreciate it." He patted his gut. "I could probably stand to lose a few pounds. I like chocolate too much."

"You might want to get a port," I said, showing him mine. "It's easier to —"

"My oncologist said I wouldn't really need one."

"So did mine, but I did. And I was glad I did. You should look into one."

My presence disturbed him. My words frightened him. Her was shutting down. I backed off.

I wheeled my Tower of Power to the bathroom and lied, "Oh, you'll do fine."

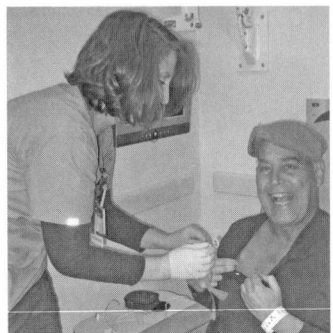

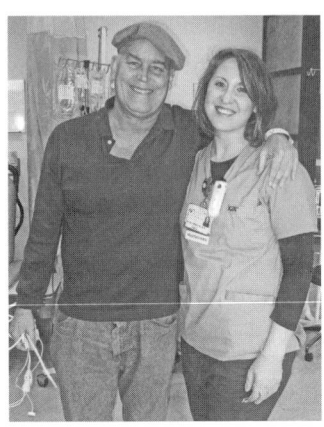

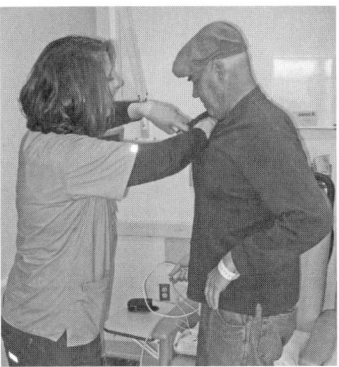

My last day of chemo! It's a big day. Wouldn't be great if hospitals did exit interviews, then gave you a nice card signed by the oncology nurses? Come on guys, *something* for the effort!

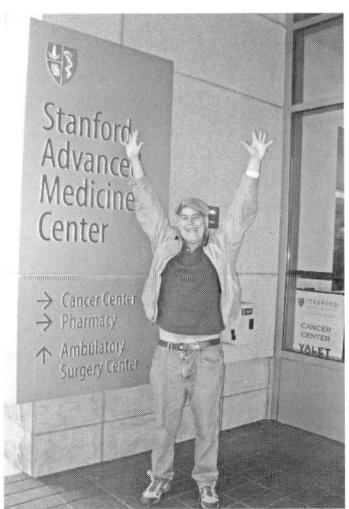

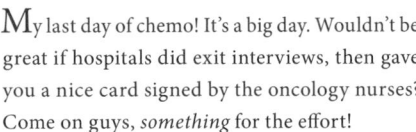

"YOU'RE DONE," SAID JANET, MY ONCOLOGY NURSE, GENTLY NUDGING ME. I woke up. I lowered my shirt collar. She unsnapped the Huber needle from my port. I laugh. I was *released*. "This is a big day."

"Hard to believe it's over," I said. "You know what might be a good idea? If on someone's last day of chemo, they get a card to congratulate them signed by all the oncology nurses. Hey, this is my Last Day of Chemo. It's like graduation. I suffered for months and months."

It was weird. The last day and now, nothing! I was just cut loose. No exit interview. It was like coming back from a war and no parade.

"I still have to go through an operation." I stood up. "Then a PET scan to see if there's any cancer left in me."

"You're not coming back here," said Janet, smiling. "*I know it.* You've done everything so well. I've seen a lot of people and you're going to make it."

"Thank you," I said, tearing up. "Can I get a hug?"

And she hugged me and I let the tears roll.

I glanced at the new recruit in a recliner, contentedly receiving his chemo through an IV in his arm, eating a graham cracker, sipping grape juice and reading a magazine. He was under the misconception that every step in his treatment could be calibrated and managed. He had no clue that in a few weeks, everything he believed would soon be shredded by a sawed-off shotgun double-barrel blast of chemical-tinged razor-blade-edged steel ribbons.

It was checkout time. I stopped at the oncology nurse station. I brought them some going-away presents. A few staffers were at the desk. I admired these women. I owed so much to these nurses. They are the curing force that makes drugs more effective. The nurses didn't let judgments of people interfere with their duties — *they only saw the pain.* They were my travel guides, Sherpas, sounding boards, bodyguards, and nutritionists. These nurses *dealt* with cancer patients and held chemo. They *cared* for the patients, spent time with them, listened to them, tried to relieve suffering — and bullshitted the difficult ones. *They see too much.* No wonder nurses have a reputation as hard partiers! Yet their opinions and feedback are often ignored by oncologists. We were cases the oncologist interpreted through scans and test results, but to the nurses we were people with emotions and lives. Not once in the four weeks did I see an oncologist talking to a nurse or like I said before, even a patient. I'm not saying it didn't happen, I'm just saying I never saw it. They only had to walk up one floor!

"Hey I brought something for you guys," I said, opening my gym bag and pulling out books, DVDs and chocolate malt protein drinks. "Here are the protein drinks I *never* ever want to drink again." The nurses laughed. "I know the drinks are expensive, give them to someone else. I thought they might help somebody." I paused. "Not only will I never drink those things again. I'll never want to eat fucking graham crackers or drink apple juice ever." They laughed. "Here are some books that helped me, and I thought they might help you guys or the patients. This one's by comedian Robert Schimmel, *Cancer on $5 (Chemo Not Included),* and this one is a wonderful book of people talking about battling cancer, *We The Victors.* It's the best one I ever read. I bought a bunch of them. Here are some DVDs I burned of *The Doctor,* a film, where a callous surgeon gets cancer and has to go through the hospital experience and learns about humanity."

"I've heard of this film," said a nurse. "The doctors should see these too."

"That's why I'm giving you a bunch of them." I paused. "So many people like me go through chemo, and nobody's here. No one to take down the foods I was able to eat to make it easier on the next patient? Or the pain relief I needed during chemo? And ports, what about having a port? That's so huge, it's just so huge."

"Tell that to the people up top, we can't," replied a nurse.

"I will do that. I'll write a letter." I paused. "Thanks so much for what you did for me." I walked away, and added. "You guys are great and oncologists are dicks!"

I got a huge laugh.

Finally, a room I can work. And I'm leaving. Hope I don't get a return engagement. Knock wood, right? And everything else.

WHEN I GOT HOME, A WIDE STRIP OF TAPE WAS STRETCHED ACROSS THE OPENING OF OUR GATE. I broke through the ribbon to the finish line of my chemo marathon. I paused at the top of the stairs to our home. Laurie and my caregivers are standing below on the deck cheering and applauding. *I'm here.* The life I built has an unobstructed view. So far, I have a privileged chance to see it — again. I descend three flights of stairs hearing my high notes of grateful and thankful for the unpredictable guardian angels who came out of the wilderness and gave me the most valuable thing in life: *their time.* They were my reinforcements whose support and love multiplied and divided faster than the hauntingly clear cancer cells that tried to obscure, blacken and devour me. In my fight against cancer, they gave me an extra knuckle on my fist. All I could do was hang my head, sniffle and blink. I enjoyed the feel around me. Good people never let you go away *unless you leave with something.* That's why love always sticks and builds. Maybe that's why it never occurred to me to give up. I didn't know how to. I had too much of this. I never wanted to leave here.

"Great," I joked, sitting down among the celebrants. "Some party, I sit here and watch you eat food and drink wine and beer I can't taste."

And they complimented me: "I was so proud of how you went through everything."…"You were an inspiration."…"Not once when I drove you to the hospital did you complain, you looked at everything you were going through as a way to get better."…"You were brave."

There's Laurie. *And they say I'm the brave one?* Throughout my chemo gauntlet she supported me. She went to the drugstore for my medications. Laid out vitamins. Kept me hydrated with energy drinks, tea, instant breakfasts. Every day she scoured grocery shelves for food and popsicles she thought my chemo palette might taste — and sometimes she broke down crying in the aisles. When I shivered in bed she layered blankets and her warm body on me. She purchased thicker sweatpants and a knit cap to keep me even warmer. *And they say I'm the brave one?* What about the doctors and nurses who called me at home, inquired about my care, suggested medications or alternatives? *And they say I'm the brave one?* The caregivers who offered themselves as my body shield in a chemo-cancer crossfire. They drove me to treatment and did everything to alleviate my suffering and hid their tears when I was in pain. They hugged me, held my hand, kissed me and looked into my eyes with deep concern. They gave up a sunny day or making money to bring me food, snacks, magazines, books, CDS, juices, DVDS, soups, and ensured the doctors and the nurses were aware of my needs. How many times did I see a frail, bald Chemosabi struggling and a distraught person supporting their arm or bringing them medication or water, assisting them in or out of a car, or looking up from their magazine and mournfully staring at their husband or wife or family member or friend or child, who are passed out and receiving chemo? *And they say I'm the brave one?* How do people raise us to such quiet triumphant heights? The ones who find you wherever you are. The ones who will never leave you behind. They don't parachute out. They stand by you to pull you out of your dive. It was impossible for me to completely sink in despair because all these people surfaced to float me. And after you go through chemo, they cheer and applaud and say you inspired them! *They are the brave ones. They are the inspiring ones.*

"You're my hero, what you did was heroic," said a friend.

"How can I be heroic when so many people were fighting for me?" I replied. My words catch in my throat. I cough an "eh" sound, sniff, and start crying. "How can I take the credit because everyone's love and caring really beat The Big C for me?" I sighed. "I'm not through this yet. Soon I won't have any testicles."

"Yes," said a friend, then warmly adding, "But we *still* have you."

You can be alone, beat cancer and survive. But you can't defeat cancer alone and have a life.

DEMATERIALIZED FOREVER

I **WAS DEMATERIALIZED BY CHEMO.** But a month after my last cycle, particles partially beamed back matter into my familiar and flawed shape. My allergies returned. My urine no longer smelled like sour apple cider. I regained poundage. Gas and ingestion didn't linger in the middle of my chest. It drifted to my stomach. My head felt like it had more air bubbles than bubble wrap around it. And between fading flecks of chemo's tin-foil spices in my meals, my taste was returning in tantalizing patches in much the same way your vision gradually gets restored after being zapped with a flash bulb. Hair peppered-up my scalp. Whiskers stubbled my chin. My legs itched because hair is growing. It's a second puberty. But this is a puberty I can handle because over time I learned gun control. This male awakening was a lot different for Fred-13, getting up with a morning boner pressed under his chin that threatened to take him hostage unless he met its demands. During my teenage sprawl, Fred-13 along with his erected peers destroyed plastic models we built before puberty, either blowing Revell WWII airplanes up with firecrackers, incinerating AMT classic cars with gas to melt them, or shattering Aurora horror figures apart with BB-guns. We were destroying the evidence of our childhood as part of our tribal transformation into another creature. Every Saturday we'd turn the TV to Channel 11 and watch monster movies on *Chiller Theater*. The dial only had 13 channels and a separate VHF knob for other channels that never worked (I still don't know what that knob was there for.). Our puberty-pronged support group watched tons of creature features: *Curse of The Hideous Sun Demon*, *The Four Skulls of Jonathan Drake*, *War of The Colossal Beast*, *Attack of The Crab Monsters*, *The Brain From Planet Arous*. We never tired of monsters chasing large breasted women. We related. Our bodies were werewolfing. Bring on the goo, the screams! When people get older they don't fear the dark, they're more afraid of what they see when they turn on the light! My lights are on 24-hour surveillance. I was growing hair because the monster inside me was dying.

But parts of me weren't materializing.

My ears were ringing. Fatigue warped me. My legs were stiff, as if they were encased in metal tubes. I falsely assumed it was a muscular problem and I was out of shape. But for the next several days I experienced longer intervals of intermittent balancing problems, dragging heaviness, and flashing sharp pains, which spread and didn't recede. It soaked into me, weighing me down. My feet and hands had varying and unpredictable stages of numbness. Sometimes my hands stiffened and prickled with splinters that resembled frostbite. At various times my fingers had difficulty flexing and bending, as if they were in thick starched gloves. I fumbled picking change up from the table, opening a jar, pinching a pill out of a bottle, or buttoning my shirt, and often hit the wrong keys when I typed on the computer or tried to text on my cell phone. The spaces of flesh between each bending joint of my fingers as well as the soles of my feet were like cardboard. Each of my toes felt like they were crinkling inside tiny paper bags. Sometimes when I tried to walk my legs felt like I was struggling through high snowdrifts. Other times, like I was walking on electrified gravel. Or my feet felt like partially deflated tires and I couldn't push off to get enough traction. Or a foot would lag, stick to the ground and I'd trip over myself. If I wore sandals, they'd slip off my feet and I didn't realize it until I looked down. When I was barefoot, I felt I was wearing shoes two sizes too small or still had on socks and when I curled my toes the bottoms of my feet felt like they were varnished or crackled like their surface was coated with the icing of a callous-patterned Dutch Crunch bread. The sides of my feet occasionally turned to marble. I was worried about falling. I learned to respect railings and fear stairs.

What were these unwanted guest appearances of *new* side effects?

One day, when I stood in line at the pharmacy to pick up a prescription, I dropped my keys, cautiously bent down on one knee, picked the keys up, and slowly rose by holding onto the lower shelf of a counter.

A guy in his seventies chuckled and said, "You get up like me!" I explained my numbness. He replied, "That's neuropathy. Older people like me get it."

I shrugged and said, "Well, I guess I caught up to you."

> **Neuropathy:** nerve damage, usually to the peripheral nerves in the hands, feet, arms, and legs. Chemotherapy is toxic to nerve cells. When nerves stop working, the result is tingling, numbness, weakness, and pain, even an impaired sense of touch. Neuropathy occurs when the outer sheathing or the myelin (protective covering) of nerve cells degenerate. Without this protection electrical signals are not transferred properly like if you stripped the covering off of the electrical wires. If possible, *before beginning chemotherapy*, ask if it's one likely to cause neuropathy, request amifostine. Recent studies show calcium and magnesium, or given intravenously as part of hydration during chemotherapy, can help prevent neuropathy. Oral does of glutamine have been effective in some cases. This is also worth discussing with the doctor ahead of time.

I TALKED TO A "TRIAGE" ONCOLOGY NURSE AT THE STANFORD CANCER CENTER. I was puzzled about neuropathy. Our conversation went like this:

> **Me:** But I thought chemo only goes after rapidly reproducing cells in the body. The stomach for nausea. Saliva in the mouth for sores. Hair loss. Weight loss. Cancer cells. That's all I heard about over and over.
> **Triage Oncology Nurse:** That's correct.
> **Me:** What does that have to do with nerves in my legs and hands and ears?
> **Triage Oncology Nurse:** (*Lowers voice and chillingly replies.*) Chemo? (*Pause.*) It goes after *everything*.
> (*Horror STING music.*)

One doctor told me it takes a year to get over chemo's effects. Ever light a fuse? You know how it burns through and just leaves a black streak of ash? Chemo lights the top of your head and burns through your body the same way and it takes a long time for everything to grow back. I researched more about neuropathy and uncovered upbeat nuggets like "some chemo drugs cause damage to *peripheral* nerves and in some cases it may be irreversible and never diminish in intensity." Now you tell me! Color me informed with a useless crayon. Yet another bonus point to rack up on Dr. Sri Lanka's lack-of-patient-care tote board. Obviously she isn't the only one suffering from nerve damage. When you're diagnosed with cancer, your life has a hit-and-run collision at What The-Hell-Happened? Boulevard and Where-Am-I? Road. There are no air bags to cushion you. You experience a cartwheeling concussion, stun-clotted, unable to think effectively because of shock waves rumbling through your nervous system. Yet, you're still expected to ask pertinent questions about side effects and preventative medications. *Shouldn't the oncologist at the scene of the accident have the responsibility to care for you?* Since I never even heard the word "neuropathy," let alone its meaning, how can I request glutamine, amifostine, calcium or magnesium as part of my hydration during chemotherapy to potentially lessen its effects? An exam isn't a pop quiz. It's the oncologist's job to give me the answers not test me. And "peripheral?" My finger tips and toes aren't peripherals! *They're my hands and feet!* I need them. Why is it people with all their feelings intact are so insensitive to the pain of others? Answer: Because they've been numb their entire lives.

I CAN FOCUS ON SENTENCES WITHOUT THE WORDS SMEARING IN STREAKING SKIDS ACROSS THE PAGE. Soul-wrestling against cancer's slippery hold drew me closer to a deeper uncritical appreciation for any creation, but on the flip, it also made some books, plays and films repellent to me. And why?

Because I spent hours and hours under house arrest in a recliner watching chemo drip, trying to maintain as I cautiously stepped on the unraveling end-to-end high wire of my life line that stretched across a vast emptiness opening below to engulf me. The line stayed taut from the force of a human bond and was wound tighter by all my cancer tears, thickening it, making it stable. I get infuriated by that chasm of dreamless emptiness that manipulates art and demeans the value and significance of that precious human connection that kept me in balance.

After surviving testicular cancer the first time, Fred-27 decided to see more shows in New York. I saw *Night Mother* on Broadway. The drama centers on a dysfunctional mother-daughter relationship. The conflict: daughter wants to commit suicide and the mother tries to give her a reason to live. At the end of the play, their relationship can't be healed. The daughter says, "Night, mother," goes into a room and blows her brains out. I looked at the theatergoer sitting next to me and said in disgust, "I spent $65 to find out life isn't worth living."

In George Orwell's novel 1984, Winston Smith is tortured by a totalitarian regime ruled by Big Brother. Under interrogation, his rebel spirit is broken because he betrays his lover to save himself. He's reduced to a worshipping automaton of the dictator. Orwell had tuberculosis but he never had cancer. If Orwell did, Smith would have despised a system that drove him to betray his lover. He'd conceal his hatred to get released, and go underground and become a terrorist to overthrow Big Brother. That's what a *living* person would do.

During chemo, I watched 50/50, a movie about a young guy with cancer. It was tough to see a character go through a same process. There were so many things the plot left out, and granted it's a Seth-Rogan-driven movie, but infusion patients don't bond that quickly during chemo — I mean, it's not like the bar in *Cheers* ("Hey nurse, see that brunette in the recliner? Her next round of Cisplatin is on me. So nurse, what are your vital signs? Me, I'm Scorpio with PSA rising. Say, are you in remission or are you just glad to see me?") The nurses told me they daily process seventy patients through infusion. Chemosabis come in on different schedules, and you might see a familiar face for two days, then not see them again for three weeks. And in 50/50, outside of puking, and getting his head shaved, the character has no difficulty eating, or other side effects. There's no mention of insurance not covering different treatments or frustration with doctors or a respectful nod to the nurses who do the real work. And even worse, the guy seemed to only have one friend and no one from work or his life sends him Get-Well cards or offers him rides. He doesn't question his life, *only what he hasn't done for himself*. If he only had one true friend, he should have wondered why. With the exception of the film's depiction of an uncaring oncologist, when it comes to the cancer experience, I can't say 50/50 is 50/50 — more like 10/90: 10 percent right. 90 percent stupid.

Some people critically laud 'fully realized" high art when two opposing views cancel out and you're left with the ineluctable mystery of existence. *Oooh, there are no answers only questions.* Duh. I've always hated that moment in Ibsen's *Peer Gynt* where the protagonist peels an onion to find the answer to life and ends up with nothing. You can't peel life away down to nothing. It's sticky. It laughs. It judges you. It embarrasses you. It unleashes you. You know why you peel an onion down to nothing? So you can use it as a topping for a cheeseburger.

I tried to get a better handle on my experience by reading a couple books about death and cancer: Randy Pausch's *The Last Lecture,* about his views on life as he was dying from incurable pancreatic cancer; Christopher Hitchens's *Mortality* on esophageal cancer that took his life; and, Lance Armstrong's *It's Not The Bike.* The famous cyclist's book is tainted by recent revelations of his doping to achieve seven Tour de France victories. Ironically, Lance beat cancer the same way he cheated to win bike races: Erythropoietin, known as EPO, a performance-enhancing drug to boost his blood count. *He cheated with what cured him.* He didn't learn his lesson: when you self-worship you miss the blessing at mass. Lance is a lying carnivorous bully. A post-graduate chemo thug. No wonder Armstrong got testicular cancer. The guy's a dick! Pausch approached his cancer experience like a college course and wrote a master's thesis. There are some touching moments in Pausch's book, but it seems appropriate Pausch specialized in Human Computer Intereaction, teaching students to wear goggles and create digital virtual-reality computer worlds. He viewed his cancer experience the same way. There's an hermetic campus tinge in the prose. At one point, Pausch advises the best way to avoid potential lifestyle problems is always carrying $200 on you. It's that simple, huh? *He wasn't living in the real world while he was living in the world!* No wonder he loved teaching! Pausch's approach avoided cancer's real terror the way he ducked the offer to take an animation job at Disney, and retreated to continue his childhood by teaching within the enabling protective robed arms of academia. And Hitchens? His main hook: will an atheist turn to God on his deathbed? Who the hell wants to die intact? His book lacks soul — *the soul of survival.* Throughout the slim volume, Hitchens's brain does fingertip push-ups but the words are cold chunks of coal without the diamond-generating heat of passion. He archly dismisses the two-edged serum of chemo as a "transparent bag of poison," which is technically true without cancer, its malignant dance partner. Hitchens refers to cancer as a "malady." Talk about sounding British! People in Jane Austen novels have maladies! Cancer is a word that defines itself all too well. When faced with death, steroid-frontal-lobed Hitchens ducks for cover in the trench-like folds of his cerebral cortex stating "as often as I am encouraged to 'battle' my own tumor, I can't shake the feeling that it is the cancer that is making war on me." He's a victim? Hitchens is making a major concession to the disease. This from a guy who supported the Iraq War! At another point, to illustrate cancer's randomness, Hitchens deconstructs the phrase: How can this happen to me? And foully states: "To the dumb question 'Why me?" the cosmos barely bothers to reply: Why not?" What kind of thought is that? It's a font-leaden horror. Would he say that quip to a parent as their six-year old child receives chemo? His defeatist attitude gets worse. "I sometimes wish I were suffering in a good cause, or risking my life for the good of others, instead of just being a gravely endangered patient." What about fighting for the love of others? Caring for the suffering around you? Widening your heart beyond your chest cavity? Hitchens described chemo as receiving a "transparent bag of poison" in a "venom sack" plugged into your arm that "swamps you with passivity and impotence" where you are "dissolving in powerlessness like a lump of sugar in water." Powerless during chemo, no way! *You're only powerless if you don't have access to chemo, radiation or any treatment.* And "passivity?" There's nothing "passive" about shaving your head, wearing tubes, and lugging yourself into treatment. Passivity is *refusing* treatment. I saw many courageous men, women, and children persevere through chemo. There was nothing passive about them! Or their caregivers! When you allow a nurse to access a port or stick a needle in your vein you're *involved*. I wonder if an atheist is also person who lacks faith in being redeemed through the love of others?

I couldn't watched any wildlife footage in documentaries where an animal kills another animal. It gives me cancer flashbacks. On the TV show *60 Minutes*, featured a husband-wife filmmaking team in Africa. In one film clip, a snarling pride of lions ganged up on a lone elephant in the night. A steady onslaught of growling and snarling cats leaped and swarmed over every part of the pachyderm's body to drop this majestic creature to its knees. The cats clambered on the elephant's back and fiercely clawed and tore deep gouges in its hide. I got mega-worked up watching this ferocious ambush. *I could feel each swiping paw violently slicing through my body.* Suddenly, the lions became the onslaught of cancer cells jumping me, trying to tear me apart from the inside out to take me down. I became that helpless elephant. All I could do was stay focused and walk through the ambush. I couldn't bear to see the gory feast's finale.

"No, I can't watch this, I can't watch this!" I shouted to Laurie, who was sitting near me. I bolted up, ran downstairs, sat in my room and shivered and cried. What kind of sick people film that shit? I angrily thought. Like it's news lions attack elephants. The filmmakers dismissed interceding to prevent the carnage of the innocent by simply stating those are the laws of the jungle. Fine, I thought, but will you feel that way *when the jungle takes you!* That's why I had a hard time with Pausch and Hitchens and Armstrong too. I didn't hear life-rending screams of protest against suffering in the vast emptiness of the jungle.

What can I say? Cancer converted me into a lion-eating zebra in remission who wants to protect the elephants among us. And if any predator stealthily crept towards the elephants and me, I guarantee you one thing, when you hear the screams, they're not going to be ours, it'll be the dying cries of whatever was foolish enough to attempt to take us out.

DURING CHEMO, I DIDN'T HAVE A SINGLE NIGHTMARE. I guess when your life's a nightmare, there's no room left for nightmares in your dreams. But the day before I was scheduled for my CT scan to discover if the tumor had grown or was dead, I was jarred awake three times by dark cancer-related fantasies:

> **Nightmare One**: I'm driving on a winding mountain road. Slowly, the road becomes narrower and narrower and completely disappears beneath me. My car flies into the ocean. The car sinks. I climb out and swim. I'm nowhere near the surface and out of air and realize I wasn't going to make it. I screamed, "This is a dream, wake up! Wake up!" And I did.
>
> **Nightmare Two**: I see a white fuzzy relaxed male figure reclining comfortably on a curved chair in the darkness. The man slumps over, falls and dies. I wake up. Did this mean I was dying or was it a good dream that meant the tumor in my body died instead of me? I wasn't sure.
>
> **Nightmare Three**: I'm naked and clasping the silver, steel-flat square surface of a jagged-edged golden stone column rising from the depth of a deep granite canyon. The column is one of many. The gaps between each one correspond to my height. I spring from one column to the next one, desperately grasping the sharp edge of its flat surface, then hop to another column. I wake up. Was this what my life would be like forever? Leaping from one second after second on my biological clock, knowing I could slip and fall between the seconds and lose it all?

FOR MORAL SUPPORT, I BROUGHT MY BOXING GLOVES TO THE CT SCAN. Cancer's shadowy nub of a finger on my eye's lens that prevented a clear view of life was gone. I was snapped back into focus. Instead of feeling removed from my life by being here, today is the first time I felt detached from the hospital's surroundings — they receded. *I was no longer of this.* Before, I was out of balance. I didn't feel all of me because I sensed there was presence inside me. The heavy hollowness that drifted through my body had vanished. My flesh no longer held me in custody. All I felt was gratitude to the nurses and doctors and friends who cared for me. That made me feel even healthier because cancer is incapable of gratitude — it's never satisfied.

After I changed into a hospital gown, the radiology attendant escorted me into a room for the CT scan. She was amused at the boxing gloves on my hands.

"I don't want you to think I'm a pyscho or something, but I've been bringing these gloves with me because I don't want to give cancer the impression I'm not fighting it. My fight's got to happen from the outside in and the inside out."

"I think that's great," she said, smiling. "Fantastic." She took photos of me. "Your oncologist will get the results of the scan right after we do them."

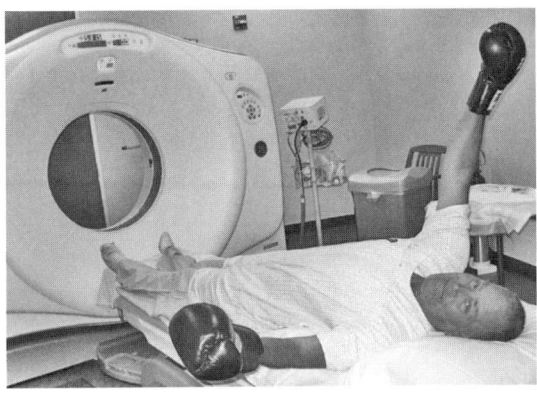

How many people pose for a picture that will tell them if you're going to live or die? *Get angry at cancer not your situation.* You gotta go in gloves up!

"I have an appointment with her after this," I said, posing with upraised gloves.

The attendants went into their lead-lined control room to microwave me. I was on my back on a tray and mechanically slid into the front-loading scanner. The white clinical cylinder whirred around me. Tears rolled out of me like sweat. Cancer's gravity demands moisture. If the scan shows iodine has located a blood source by a form that's not an organ, the tumor is still feeding.

My voice cracked as I whispered to the potential horror of a sprawling latency, "You're not here, you're not here."

The Big C is a potential predator for the rest of my life. It's part of me. Then again, so were the fillings in my teeth.

LAURIE AND I WAIT IN THE EXAMINATION ROOM OF CLINIC E TO GET THE RESULTS OF MY CT SCAN. I hope this is my final appointment with the personality-challenged Dr. Sri Lanka. She popped through the door like one of those antique clock wood-carved figures announcing the hour.

"I have good news for you," Dr. Sri Lanka says, smiling. "The CT scan shows your tumor has gone from 22 centimeters to 3. What's left is probably dead tissue or benign. Your last PET scan shows some glowing in the tumor area. We feel those cancer cells are dying. The tissue is on your iliac vein and would require you to undergo major surgery. We'd rather wait to see if the cancer is dead than perform that surgery."

I must face the killer who turned my body into a crime scene.

"Can I see the tumor?"

She nodded and replied, "Certainly."

We go into another room that has students in lab coats working at various desks. Dr. Sri Lanka inserted a disc into a computer drive. The screen fills with gray and white throbbing blotches. She sifts through them and identifies various organs, but to me, the whole thing looks more like a black-and-white x-ray of a dirty martini. Then Dr. Sri Lanka attempted something she never did before. She tried to supportively pat me, but it was more of a poke with the tip of her fingers. She pulled it back as quickly as she offered comfort, as if any form of human contact triggered her into automatic recoil. But the real reason was, she probably sensed I was repulsed from her touch. It was too little, too late.

"This is the original size of the mass," she said, making a line on the screen. She flicked to another image and drew a smaller line, "This is what it is now."

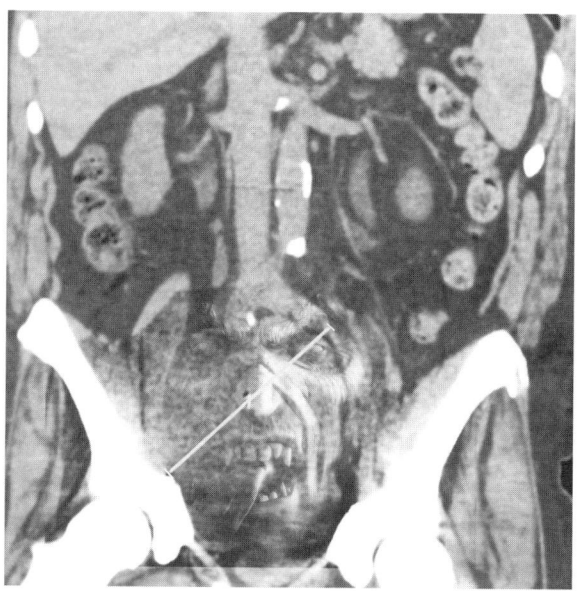

CANCER MUG SHOT: DECEMBER 2011

TUMOR ARRESTED – (Stanford Cancer Center, Palo Alto) Cancer in custody. The kidney-shaped tumor has been booked at four-pounds. It's the size of a large fist and resembles a political strategist's brain. Cancer began in a remaining testicle. The germ-based tumor is contained within lymph nodes, and may have attached to the iliac artery alongside the muscles in the lower pelvic region. The assailant blocked the right ureter, decreasing kidney function, which required patient to don catheter-and-urine-bag riot gear. Tumor will undergo a chemo trial of five 8-hour days for four weeks.

(Tumor width white line: four pounder.)

"So that's him," I said. The clumped tumor was a scar-tissued kebab along my iliac vein. I suspiciously peered at the dead killer inside me, as if I expected the squashed tumors to move. It didn't. "That's what's left *in* me."

Dr. Sri Lanka expected me be exultant. But, I was emotionally drained. I felt like a sapped penitent at the end of a pilgrimage. I'd expended all my energy to generate a force-field to resist cancer. When I it gone, I collapsed from the effort. I snapped the line, but still couldn't spit out the hook. I've taken a hit. I'm wary. I suspect a trap. The Big C might be a sniper trying to draw me into the open to waste me. I'm not an easy coax. I remain cautiously reserved out of respect. I can't drop my arms completely — ever. It's the only way of ensuring my survival.

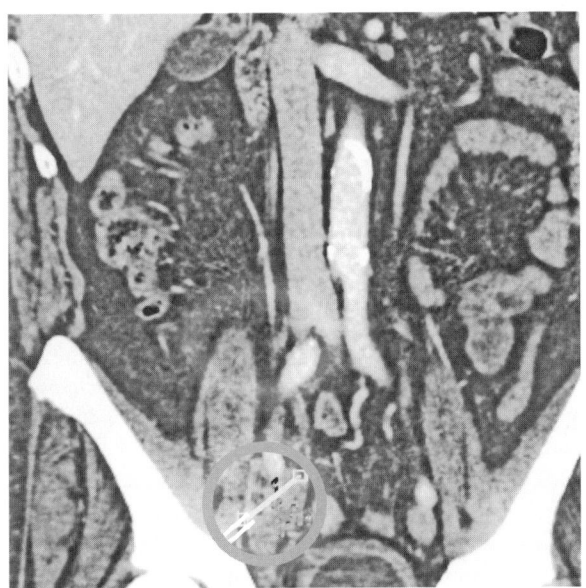

CANCER MUG SHOT: JUNE 2012

TUMOR GETS DEATH SENTENCE – (Stanford Cancer Center, Palo Alto) After three intense months of chemo incarceration, tumor is reduced to a two-inch kidney-bean shape pinky of scar tissue, weighing a few ounces, and resembles the dead conscience of a Health Maintenance Organization CEO. Ureters are unblocked. Cancer could possibly appeal the diagnosis, if a PET scan reveals tumor has signs of life, the patient may undergo a complex, life-threatening operation that will treat the tumor like its an aneurysm, and iliac vein will be clamped, cut, and resectioned. Patient has refused to give cancer a reprieve or pardon.

(*Scar tissue remains in white line within circle: a couple ounces.*)

Dr. Sri Lanka and I leave the room and stand in the hallway. We are opposite each other. Our arranged clinical marriage has ended. Cancer is the only thing we had in common. Her treatment was correct but without any support and care from her, I had to fight to relieve my pain. That really pissed me off. I had nerve damage might that have been prevented or lessened by introducing minerals to my chemo. That pissed me off. Our relationship was on a pay-as-you-go basis. I paid and now it was time for her to go. *I wondered how she would handle being sick.* I noticed her stomach had signs of stretch marks. Was she a warm mother or childless and fat? A supportive wife? No idea. She never discussed her life, or why she became an oncologist. And she never expressed any interest in my personal life! I didn't have any problems with her treatment, just how she treated me. She never saw beyond my premorbid condition — but if that's how I viewed myself during treatment, I'd be dead.

There was an uncomfortable silence between us which I enjoyed. She was expecting me to gulp emotional thank yous, impulsively hug her. *She wanted an emotion she never gave me.* No way. She had blown too many cues. I saved my gratitude for the people who cared for me. I made an attempt to mentor her in People Skills 001 in an effort to help prevent future harm to her patients.

I lied, "You know, I'm not saying you didn't care about me." Then delicately added, "But, when I was home, I would have appreciated getting a call."

"About your treatment?" she asked, puzzled.

She still didn't get it.

"Not my treatment, just a call at home to *see how I was feeling*. Or maybe if once you checked up on me in infusion when I was getting chemo. Asking how I was feeling would have showed you cared. And when a doctor shows they care, it makes the patient feel better. It's therapeutic. I'll go off on a tangent. Congressman Tip O'Neill was the Speaker of the House many years ago, but when he first ran for office and won, a woman in his old neighborhood came over to him and said, 'You never visited me but I still voted for you.' He was surprised and replied. 'But you've known me my whole life.' Then she said, 'People like to be asked.' It's kinda like that, only we want someone to ask how we are."

Dr. Sri Lanka's eyes sparked. I briefly saw the woman behind the ceramic tribal caste. It didn't last long. She was professionally indignant about not getting a thank you. She went into clinical overdrive sauteed with her unique touch of insensitive precision, "Your red blood cell count is low and we want to give you a transfusion so when you finally get over all the chemo you'll regain your strength for the operation, which will be in about a month to remove your testicle. It's necessary for the testicle to be removed. Its hormonal production has been known to stimulate tumor growth." It seemed like she wanted to upset me. Like it was a power she held over me. "In three months we'll do a PET-scan which will determine if we will have to operate to remove the tumor."

It's still not over, I thought, *after all this, it's still not over.*

Dr. Sri Lanka clearly expected me to shake her hand and say thank you. I said nothing and kept my hands in my pockets. The slighted oncologist turned on her hard flat shoes and walked away.

I asked, "I think I'm having hearing problems. Is that common?"

Without glancing back, she indifferently clipped, "Yes, chemo does that."

I *heard* that. I shook my head. Maybe, after I leave here, I should ask the hospital to solicit donations to harvest a heart for her — a human one.

I'd never see Dr. Sri Lanka again. She handed me off to another oncologist, Dr. Russell Pachynski. I didn't know if that was the normal procedure because I completed chemotherapy, or she wanted to get rid of me, but I wasn't complaining. Dr. Pachynski, turned out to be a considerate, bright, direct, responsive, and quick to get me my results. Much later, I learned Dr. Sri Lanka told another oncologist she chose oncology/urology because "men are quiet when I talk to them, don't questioned me and they do everything I tell them to do." *So, that's why she didn't like to be challenged!* Who could blame her? Women get treated badly in India. Oncology is probably a tough field for a woman. I met my share of male Stanford-educated pedigree doctors diagnosed with terminal arrogance too. But it wasn't okay to treat me the way she did. I didn't date her in India, and I wasn't an chauvanistic oncologist. Perhaps, she was conflicted because years ago *she* also lost both her testicles to cancer. My guess if she didn't, if she had a husband, he lost *his* after marrying her. Still, all I could say is I felt her anger. And when you're going through chemo and cancer, you know one thing: *you know how you feel*. I believe disagreeing with her helped me get the care I deserved, as well as experience less pain, but if I had completely submitted to her will, I'd have suffered more, and possibly gotten so depressed I might have given cancer a crucial advantage. I couldn't afford that. It still angered me. I decided to write a letter complaining about her behavior to the hospital, perhaps it might reluctantly force her to be more attentive to the next poor slob. If she didn't like it too bad. It might make her worse: a dog never likes getting their nose stuck in their own poop — especially if it's Stanford poop. Later, when I cited my unpleasant experiences with off-the rack oncologists, people who have never had cancer, propounded, "I'd rather have a great doctor with no people skills, then one with people skills who isn't a great doctor." I said, "You can also be a bad doctor with no people skills." They'd nod and say, "True." So what's their frigging point? The real deal: there's no excuse for not having compassion. But it's amazing how many people easily flee from it with a paycheck.

After my appointment, Laurie and I go back to the car and exit the hospital's garage. We stop at a gate. It six dollars for parking. It's free for 45 minutes. Who the hell can get an examination in 45 minutes? Why don't they make it two hours? Why should my car have a copay?

I hand the money to the attendant and said, "I guess having cancer isn't good enough to validate parking."

The attendant ignores me, he's heard it before — too bad no one is listening.

Parking wasn't free and neither was I.

Use your chemo leverage! Never be ashamed of your bald head. Whenever you can, take off your hat and ask people to kiss it for good luck. Beam your sheen!

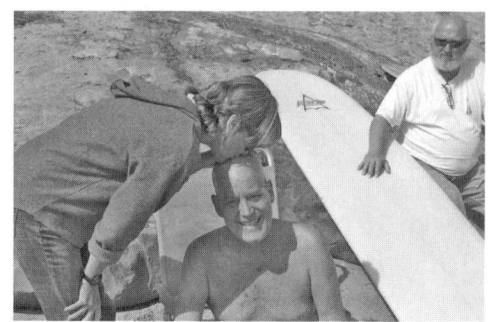

WEEKS PASSED, MY ORCHIECTOMY WAS SCHEDULED FOR TOMORROW. I wanted to hit the ocean one more time. There was a decent swell pumping through the point. The break was swarming with people. I decided not to go where the waves were breaking best. Today, my goal was to stay out of everyone's way. I'd sit off the main peak where very few waves were, hoping to catch smaller scraps surfers either missed or didn't want.

Driveway Dave was in the cove below the rocks of the cliff, chucking a tennis ball for Blake. He spotted me and said, "Hey Fred, I know you want to go out, but only after I tell you something, then I'll shuttup."

Dave loved to talk. If you didn't initiate the conversation, he'd introduce new topics himself, comment on them, and if you didn't respond, he'd bring up another subject and continue on and on. It was part of his charm, really

"No you won't," I replied. "You never stop talking."

"I never stop talking," he said and smiled. "Bill and Diane told me that too."

"Bill and Diane?"

"I introduced them to you."

"You introduce me to people who I don't know and I'm not sure if I will ever like. Anyone can be nice on land. It's how they act in the water. If they're nice in the water, I'll get to know them. Most of the people out there have two sides and I don't like either one. If you're on land you don't think piranhas are that bad, and if you're in the water you don't think lions are that bad. It's location, location, location. Most of these new fake-cool people out there can be lions or piranhas at the flip of a coin."

"Your operation is tomorrow, right?" said Dave, who was always expressed concern about my health. He's a caring guy.

"When they take my last testicle," I said, "I'll officially be a registered Democrat." I paused. "I'll also be able to check the box on the application that says 'Married.'"

"This is what I wanted to speak to you about," said Dave. "I hope you won't take it personal." Dave discussed my novel *Blind Guys Break 80*. He said, "Are you Cloudy? (The main character.)" I said, "Part of me." "Clear, the other character, was your Dad?" "Yes." "And that part of being from Freehold, New Jersey, and then having to move and being in a new place and not fitting in? That was biographical?" "Yes." Dave said, "I had a hard time because it dealt with golf, but when I got to the part dealing with the family. You had me. There was a part…" His voice caught. "Where the mother says, 'Help me' in the hospital." He started crying. "That happened to me too." He paused. "I was real glad I bought the book."

"Well, thanks."

"And the alcoholism in the book, you nailed that. No matter what anyone tells you, never change your opinion about that. I was an alcoholic. When I was one. I didn't acknowledge that word, because saying I was an 'alcoholic' meant I had to *do something about it*. With all that drinking in your family, how come you never became an alcoholic?"

"Because I *saw* it," I said, smiling. "My sister Stephanie has been one for fourteen years. And she loves to play that self-pity violin. You'd think by now one of the strings would break. Some people hit bottom and change. But a lot of people *like* the bottom. There are a lot of people down there. I have a tough time dealing with my family now. Awhile ago, the day after Dad died, I was talking about the estate to my other sister, Cindy, who was the executor, and she said, 'No one tells me what to fucking do.' I was stunned. She's all control and drama. She won't listen to anybody."

"Yeah, my ex-wife is like that," said Dave, smirked. "She knows *everything*."

"I'd never do to my siblings what they did to me. I lost money in probate court. But you know what I inherited? The best of my Mom and Dad. And my parents' spirits throughout all I've gone through have come to me, and they're always with me, and I don't think my brother and sisters have that because all they did was look at my parents and wait for another apple to fall from the tree, but they never brought anything to the tree. What's weird is they all know and bring up when it's our parents' birthdays and anniversary. I think it's out of guilt. Stephanie said after Dad died, 'He should have taken better care of us.' Sending her to college wasn't enough! And you know what's even weirder? Not one of them seems to have any dreams about being something else beside themselves. Don't care about owning a house, having a career. Just get by, live off the grid, drink at the local bar. They don't want to get on with their lives that's fine — I have mine."

"Your brother and sisters never forgave you for leaving."

"When I was out here doing temp jobs, and struggling at stand-up comedy, if I was hungry and broke, I stayed hungry and broke. Hey, my parents helped me out once in awhile, sure. But if they had it tough, they went over to our parents' place and got money and dinner. I didn't have any unresolved issues with Mom and Dad. I never took vacations. If I had free time, I flew back to visit my folks — and being with family isn't a vacation. When I was there, my sisters said to me, 'You're the one who got everything.'" I laughed. "So Dave, can I go out in the water now and live my life?"

I paddled out and sat on my board next to The General, a 67-year old local guy who surfed this spot for many years. It was unusual to see him in the water. He had soured on the overcrowded conditions and people's rudeness. We were the only two sitting outside of the main break.

"They don't get it," said The General, pointing to the horde of beginners or whatever they were, dropping in on each other on blue foam boards. "I had a girl take off behind me, and I couldn't cutback. *She knew better.* But she acted like she didn't know. I couldn't ride my wave." He paused. "Years ago, I was surrounded by surfers, now I'm surrounded by people on surfboards."

I said, "I can't let them keep me out of the water. It means too much to me. I'm trying to get stronger. I tell Driveway Dave — "

"Dave talks to everyone. He has a good heart. Those people are using him to take from us. If they get you to say hello, it gives them access to the surf spot, then they burn you and take the waves. That's how they get through life. Takers. When I was a kid, Dad was in the army, and I made some money shining shoes and doing a lot of things, and I kept all my money in a sock I hung out my window. I told a friend of mine where I kept my money. And the next day the sock with my money was gone. It was the best thing that ever happened to me. Here I thought I was so important and special because I had money, and it was gone and I wasn't any of those things anymore. I've never trusted money since."

"When I was going through chemo there were two people inside me," I said. "There was my body pulling me down and there was this other guy inside me who was saying, 'Who are you kidding? You're not going, anywhere. You — '"

"You have seven spirits inside you," The General sagely interrupted me, pointing to his face. "There's smell, taste, sight, hearing..."

"I had only those two," I said. "But they were there."

"Those spirits heal you. They are in you," said The General as we bobbed in the ocean. "A lot of people were never taught to find them. Some of them need Jesus to do it. But that's only one spirit. I saw this TV show and these elephants came upon bones of another elephant, and they carried them in their trunks. They *knew.* I cried. There are people who don't have *that.* I knew a man who was a healer. People who were sick could talk and listen to him and he would heal them. Later in life he was very sick, and heavy because he took on their energy, it had to go somewhere, and he put it onto himself."

A phalanx of pelicans flew over us in a V-formation.

"I always wonder how pelicans decide who is the leader," I said.

"They don't have a leader, the formation keeps shifting. One moves up and another moves back with the currents, I watch them, I know." The General paused. "I'm glad I'm out here now. Talking to you like this. Before I was all upset because that girl ruined my wave. Women in the surf don't pay the dues we pay. Now they're all over the place, telling us what to do. Where were they thirty years ago? Nobody was stopping them. Why?"

I replied, "Because the guys who surfed then were misfits they didn't want to date. Now you have lawyers, doctors and career people. The water got civilized so women felt safer. They came out when they got the "all clear" signal. The boards are lighter, wet suits are warmer. Now it's like they come out here with families to meet other people. Then they tell us the new rules. The worst."

A wave finally came through.

"Let's go for it," said The General. "Share."

I started paddling, but The General was in the perfect spot. Besides, I couldn't spring up, and would only interfere with his ability to catch the wave. I didn't go. Maybe there was another wave behind it. There wasn't. I waited for a half hour. No wave came. I paddled in. I struggled in the shorebreak to the beach. Dave came out and helped me. He put my board down on the sand.

"Fred, you want to sit?" asked Dave, offering his beach chair. "Really take my chair." He paused. "Want some candy corn? A water?"

"I'm fine thanks," I said, leaning against the rocks.

"I don't know if you're an atheist or an agnostic, I don't think much about it," said Dave as we looked at the ocean. "I knew this Christian and they were all crying at someone's death and I said to them, 'Why are you crying. You should be happy because he's in a better place.' But my wife says about religion, 'Whatever people believe that's what will happen to them.' I never spent much time on it, but there's no reason not to be nice to people."

"For you maybe," I said, smiling. "Because you're desperate for anyone to talk to."

"You and I think alike."

"Can you tell what I'm thinking now?"

He smiled.

I pushed off the rocks to stand and almost fell. The muscles in my unsteady legs pulled at my joints like a dried-out rubber bands that lost their elasticity.

"Do you need help with your board?" Dave asked. "I'm here."

"I should carry it myself to get stronger," I said, then noticed my legs were still wobbling. I sighed. "I do need help."

Dave took my board up the steps from the beach. I hobbled behind him, clinging to the railing.

"Good luck tomorrow. Be happy you've got doctors who know what's wrong with you and are able to do something about it."

"Some people don't come out of anesthesia."

"Yeah, that's what people say about me," said Dave.

A muscular Stud Guy in his mid-twenties imperiously stood at the top of the stairs. He wore bright spandex workout clothes, a baseball cap and earplugs connected to an iPod. He held two enormous German Shepherds on chain leashes. He blocked us but wasn't going to move because we were in *his* way.

I smiled and said, "Hi."

Stud Guy ignored my greeting and stared at us. Instead of politely moving aside and letting us pass, the colon-brained moron stomped down the stairs, elbows out, and charged through us. His dogs brushed against our legs. Dave almost dropped my board. I lost my balance. I went ballistic. *This macho jerk is acting like I'm not here.* That's what would have happened if I died from cancer: I wouldn't be standing here. I'm not dead! I'm alive and this jerk is going to know it. I don't care how big he is, or if his dogs are mean. *I'm alive, fuck him.*

I furiously spewed, "Hey fuckhead, you can't return a hello from somebody because you're wearing your stupid earplugs." He turned. "When I say 'hello' you're supposed to say 'hello' back." He went down the stairs. "What about an 'excuse me? You're rude. Hey, you're an asshole. You hear me, you're an asshole."

The guy kept going down the steps.

Driveway Dave shrugged and said, "What can you do? It is what it is."

"No, it isn't what it isn't. I'm over it," I said. "He's his own problem. You know the difference between him and us?" I paused. "*We can be cured.*"

I enjoyed my fury. This was a warning sign of something else, I had to overcome but I didn't recognize its warning symptoms.

I DROVE AWAY FROM PLEASURE POINT. I hooked up my iPod to the radio and put on *Forever* by the Beach Boys to create a soundtrack. I looked at the world I returned to, a world where I was unhooked and liberated and beginning to taste and smell and see and live in again and I drove and smiled and images opened up to me like the light of a movie projector as a film passed over my eyes.

> *If every word I said could make you laugh*
> *I'd talk forever*

Months ago, I was in bed, shivering in my chemo curl, wondering if the film would snap and my movie abruptly end. But even as tears streaked down my face I couldn't believe I was going to die, a buoyant force pulsating from beyond was still within me and I couldn't sink and that power brought me back here with the tail of my surfboard sticking out above the windshield as I listened to the Dennis Wilson plaintively sing.

> *If the song I sang to you*
> *Could fill your heart with joy I'd sing forever...*

"I'm back," I said, my lips quivered as tears of inspiration reform in my eyes. Let the others call this a karmic rerun. But I love the sequels of me! I climb upon the steady pulse of an uplifting feeling and deeply inhale refreshed air. I say to The Great Unknown, "Thank you. I want to stay. Let me stay, please let me stay."

> *Let the love I have for you,*
> *Live in your heart and beat forever.*

The General never told me the names of the seven spirits. But it didn't matter. All seven were going full blast.

THE NIGHT BEFORE MY ORCHIECTOMY, I WATCHED A DVD OF *THE DOCTOR*. It's a 1991 movie based on the book, *A Taste of My Own Medicine* by Dr. Edward E. Rosenbaum. After Laurie went to bed, I stayed up late to watch it again. I figured a film about cancer might upset her, so I watched it by myself.

William Hurt plays Jack McKee, an insensitive and arrogant surgeon who is diagnosed with throat cancer. McKee's illness forces him to view medicine, hospitals, and doctors from a patient's perspective. He realizes there's more to being a doctor than surgery and prescriptions. He becomes a compassionate healer. I love many scenes in this movie. One where he tells off his doctor: Oncologist: "Doctor, I know how you're feeling." McKee: "That's the problem you don't have the first idea of what I'm feeling… I think you ought to brush up your act, Dr. Abbott. Because today I'm sick, tomorrow, or the day after, or thirty years from now you'll be sick. Every doctor becomes a patient somewhere down the line, and then it'll hit you as hard as it hit me." But my favorite scene is after McKee has learned his lesson. He performs a heart transplant. In the operating room, he looks into the red opening of his patient's chest cavity and tenderly speaks, "Start beating sweet heart." The machine beeps. "Go heart." He laughs in quiet wonderment. Then he takes off his bloody surgical glove, gently strokes the sedated patient's forehead and in a comforting voice says, "It's a beautiful heart."

I had to see those scenes. I break down watching them. Then sigh, knowing tomorrow I'm going into surgery too. I needed to see the warmth from the value of life. It sustained me. The movie reinforced my courage and frightened me.

AN OMEN TERRIFIES ME. Before we leave for the operation at the hospital, I find the cactus plant on the steps below the outside deck. The Popeye Spinach can is on its side. The poor plant's leaves were wilted and faded and its upraised and clawing roots were blanched in the air atop a tiny pyramid of spilled-out dry dirt. A cat, squirrel or the wind must have knocked the cactus off the deck's railing. A bad sign. Like finding a dead baby bird that dropped from a nest at your front door. I panicked. Was the withered cactus a premonition the tumor was going to reappear in my body? If my green buddy perished and didn't bloom, I wasn't going to bloom. *I wasn't going to make it!* Or is this a sign that when they open me up today, they'll find more cancer? And then there's the chance for an infection. I sucked in my lips and thought of Dad lying in the gurney with his unshaven face and flat eyes. Was I going to die like he did?

I scooped up the dirt, and replaced the six-inch plant in his Popeye Spinach can. I put the plant in the shade because he already had enough sun. I need you to get well, I thought. But the cactus looked really wasted. I watered the little guy and softly kneaded the moist soil with my fingers tips. I can't abandon him. We had gone through chemo and cancer together. I wasn't giving up on him — or me.

WHEN FACED WITH GIVE ME TESTICLE OR GIVE ME DEATH, I GIVE UP MY RIGHT NUT FOR THE WELL-HUNG VIEW OF A NEW DAY. Laurie and I stood at the doors to the surgery waiting room. I rest my hand on the handle and utter a mmm-groan gasp. During World War II flying missions, bombardiers sat on their helmets because they were worried about getting their balls blown off. Here I am low to the ground and paying to lose what's left of mine. If I want to live everything must go. My resolve crumbles like coffee cake. Am I standing in crumbs or a forked-over crumb of a man?

As I open the door I say to Laurie, "This is as real as it gets." I wonder, will this ever end? Will this be the beginning of surgeons carving more pieces out of me? I mutter, "My life is so fucked."

The waiting room looks more like a bus terminal. It's noisy. There are families. Unattended kids running through the aisles. There are even midgets or "little people" or whatever you want to call them. I envy them, they're smaller than me, but their world is a lot bigger than mine today. There's laughter. Pockets of silence. Others doing their office work on laptops or playing games on their iPad. Rude people on cell phones next to patients who are frightened about their procedure. I register for my orchiectomy. We sit down. I pick up Laura Hillenbrand's *Unbroken*.

Laurie takes out a newspaper and whispers to me, "How can some people just sit here, and stare straight ahead and not do anything?"

"They're worried."

My cell phone rings. It's a Connecticut number. It could be my sister Stephanie, who has me on drunk-and-dial. I dread answering it.

Cancer is a dividing line. It's where you cut and share the cake. There's the stale past on one side and the future, moist and fresh on the other. Then again, there's family — and that has nothing to do with any even scale. After Dad died there were ugly scenes about money in his estate. There are two kinds of grief: 1.) The grief you have when you lose a parent or loved one. 2.) The grief your family gives you in probate court. The Big C had made me stand at the Blackboard of My Life and erase all the things I thought were once important or irritated me, but money issues don't go away: numbers remain. The money figure my siblings cost me was still on the blackboard. Repaying the debt is the only thing that will make it right. But if they were capable of doing the right thing, I wouldn't have the problem. They never dealt with reality because my parents cleaned up their messes. My siblings saw nothing wrong with living off the estate and lying to me. I realized that's how they went through life and treated other people. Why should I be any different? I was no longer a brother, I was reality and they treated me the same way.

I got up, walked down the hallway and answered the phone. It's my brother, Bill. I don't know what to say to the guy sometimes. When Dad was in the hospital, I had his wallet. Before he went into surgery, he asked me to make sure I had the oil changed in his car. I had it done. There were five bucks left in Dad's wallet. When I came back to the condo, I put the wallet down on the kitchen table and left. My brother was in the room. I came back a few minutes later. I checked the wallet. The money was gone. I said, "You know, I thought there was five dollars left in here." He stared at me, shrugged his shoulders and dumbly said, "I don't know." I didn't want to get into an accusation drama. He had to live with the act not me. What do you do with people like that? He was more intelligent than he seemed. Sometimes I wondered if the guy felt bad about anything. Our parents sent him to college and all he did was party, and has pretty lived the same routine for the next thirty years, working various jobs, getting fired or laid off, and going to bars every night. He was in his late forties, single, and collecting unemployment. He didn't seem to want anything else out of life. One time, Dad took out a second mortgage of $40,000 to help Bill start up a business, and that went up my brother's nose. None of it seemed to bother him. He only get furious if you brought the topic up. He shared one common reflex with my sisters. If you confronted them with any truth about themselves or responsibility for their actions, they either became angry, blamed you for their problems, stared and said nothing, or lied. During probate, Bill said to me, "Family has to stick together." "I don't have a family," I replied. "Family shares their troubles, after Dad died everyone just thought of themselves." "You can't tell people how to live their lives," he said. I added, "Yeah, it's a good thing Mom and Dad never felt that way, huh? They gave us everything." Weird guy. During probate I got a lawyer, Bill said he'd pay half the fees, then when he got his money he never sent me a dime. I brought it up to him. He replied, "Patience is a virtue." I said, "Then I must be the most virtuous person on earth." And left it there.

Bill said on the phone, "So what do they do to you?"

"They don't go into your sack. They make an incision in the groin above the penis and pop out the testicle by the sperm cord like a YoYo on a string, then snip the cord."

"Cindy and Stephanie want to talk to you."

"No, no, no, no!" I snap.

He hands off the phone to Stephanie.

"We're family, we have each other," Stephanie said, clearly drunk. She starts crying and whining. "I'm so upset about what you're going through. I'm really upset. I can't handle it." She coughs. "I have a cold. I think I'm allergic to bug spray. I'm having a hard time. My meds cost too much. I know I haven't called or been there for you. I'm sorry. I don't have any money. I'm so upset, I really am. But I can't handle it." I had cancer and I'm minutes away from getting my remaining testicle lopped off, but the most important and tragic thing is *she can't handle it*. I don't say anything. I didn't want drama. She lived for drama. They all did. But it only becomes a drama if you step on the stage and argue with them. Stephanie hasn't had a job in fourteen years. She's an alcoholic who lived off her divorce settlement and our parents until they died. My sister Cindy, the executor, against my wishes allowed Stephanie to live in our parent's condo rent-free and live off the estate. Cindy sold the condo at a huge loss. Stephanie moved in with Cindy and lives off them now. She gets drunk on cooking sherry or liquid hair spray and gets on the phone and dials relatives, or passes out in her room for days, and sometimes throws dishes and coffee cups at Cindy and calls her a fat pig and my brother a drunk. She passed out on a space heater and got severe second-degree burns on her leg. She explained it away saying, "I'm clumsy." It was hopeless. She wasn't really going to change until she became her own problem. Then she'd probably try to get disability and live off the state. How can I write this? Because this Thing isn't my sister. Not the girl I grew up with. Besides, if she doesn't like this, she can sober up, she has potential to be shape up, or use this as an excuse to drink, right? It's a win-win for her. It's the best I can do.

"I love you," she said.

"I'm being called for surgery," I lied. "Thanks."

She hands off the phone to Cindy. In a way, Stephanie is Cindy's karma. I have a hard time with Cindy too. Laurie and my financial straits are the result of how Cindy handled the estate to benefit herself. We almost lost our house. At the time of our Dad's death, Cindy, her boyfriend, and Bill were living in a rented apartment. I suggested they buy out my share of the condo, and wait until housing prices go up, sell the place at a profit and get on with their lives. Cindy charged, "You just want the money! What do we get?" "You get a place to live and equity." "I don't want to have a mortgage and pay taxes." I futilely suggested, "You can keep all the furniture in the place, Mom and Dad would want you to. And whatever profit you make from the condo sale later, you keep. And you get a tax break on the mortgage, and even then, it's still cheaper than the rent you're paying now." She angrily insisted, "You just want the money." I mentioned the condo deal to my brother and he replied, "I'd be too far from the bars to party." Stephanie thought the condo was hers because she was living with Dad and said, "You know why they don't want to live in the condo? Because it would be under *my* rules. I'm the one who is keeping the family together." So how did it all play out? Instead of living in the condo, they all moved into an apartment above a bar, and paid more in rent than it would have cost them to live in the condo. Laurie and I struggled to keep our house and my siblings' lives remained unaffected, living off the grid, and Cindy and her boyfriend planned a vacation. Nice. I later found out, Cindy's unemployed boyfriend, had a couple hundred thousand in the bank, which meant everything could have been a non-issue — but he *also* didn't want a mortgage or pay taxes either. And his parents also rented their entire lives. Duh! What can you say to this dysfunction junction? Point to a door to escape a fire, they'll walk back into the building, and criticize you for not trying to put out a blaze they started. There are people you can't talk to. And problems you can't solve. You can offer valid solutions and they'll still make decisions that hurt themselves — but only as long as they hurt you too. Why yell at an overflowing toilet? Family wasn't a two-way street, so I don't drive down it anymore. I had more of my share of head-on collisions, and more pressing issues.

"So what are they going to do to you?" asked Cindy, concern in her voice.

I explain the operation and my projected recovery, then lie again, "I have to go."

"I love you."

"Thanks for calling."

I was glad that was over. What can I say to my family when they did more financial and emotional harm to me than anyone else in my life? Outside of trying to cut these phone calls short, I never lied to them, and when it came to family I never stole from them. Sure, there's still a love. But it's distant. And something ends. I stopped calling them, and didn't send presents on their birthdays or Christmas. After all they're the ones who blew me off the map. But they didn't send me any either. It's harsh writing about these things. But they'll get angry for the wrong reason. They're more concerned about how other people perceive them then what they did to me. Fine, they've gotten the life they wanted, but was it worth losing a brother? Maybe. I lost a brother and two sisters. They still came out ahead.

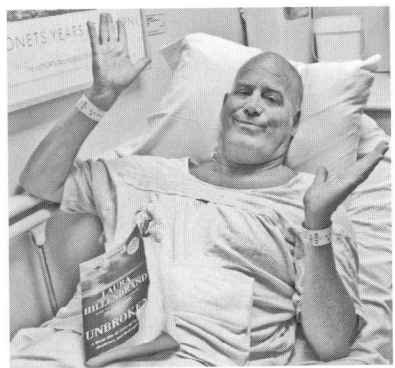

Read books about real people triumphing over adversity. Now, it's your turn to be one. Rescue yourself! Imagine what you'll be able to do to help others face this!

Radical Inguinal Orchiectomy: the surgical removal of one or both testicles, or testes, in the human male. An incision is made in the groin and the testicle is plucked out of its sack by pulling the sperm cord, through the incision, then the cord is snipped and removed.

BALLS OUT OF PLAY. Testicle Number One: (HANG TIME: 1954– 1982). And today in surgery, scheduled for lift off is Testicle Number Two: (HANG TIME: 1954 – 2012). Thanks for the ride, boys. Now, it's Radical Inguinal Orchiectomy time. Inguinal? Sounds like a spicy penne pasta dish with calamari. **An orchiectomy is a balless way saying "castration" or "emasculation."** And granted a complete testicle removal for some guys is the same as a frontal lobotomy, or for others a divorce settlement. After this surgery, if I wear a speedo, I'll be the only male on the beach showing an erection and camel toe. Perhaps I'll come out of the operation as a soprano castrato and run a amazing string of High "C" Notes.

I can't stand opera, but I'm currently unemployed and a gig is a gig. Maybe I can hire the hospital harpist to accompany me at recitals before boring overeducated rich people. Or maybe, if they ever make another film of *The Sun Also Rises*, I can be the Jacob Barnes's stunt double in the *lack* of explicit sex scenes. I looked up orchiectomy. *Orchis* is the ancient Greek word for testicle. It made me wonder if cynical Greeks made jokes about the Spartans by saying, "Have you heard the latest edict from the noble Orchis Aurelius?" And *ectomy* means "a cutting out of." I doubt if an orchiectomy was originally a surgical procedure, more likely, I bet an orchiectomy was either a battlefield tactic, an early feminist movement launched by Sappho, or a highly effective take-down move by gladiators. As far as I'm concerned, *orchis* means "spay" and *ectomy* means "neutered." It's difficult to register how the surgery will affect me. Will I overcompensate not having testicles the way women deal with being small breasted? If I go out, will I wear a padded, push-up athletic supporter? Or date one?

Before I'm admitted for my orchiectomy, I must undergo a non-medical mandatory procedure or I'll be denied surgery: I must sign a waiver. But it's not called a "waiver." It's a *consent form*. Legally how do they get away with this? But it's accepted extortion. What will they do if I don't sign it, cut my balls off? I "consented" to get nephrostomy tubes, CT/PET scans, biopsies, chemotherapy and now, an orchiectomy. What do these "consents" have in common? Answer: They absolve the doctors from any consequences of their diagnosis and *I assume all the risks*. When they graduated and were asked to take the Hippocratic oath did they say, "Under advice of my attorney, I refuse to make any statements that may incriminate myself in the future."? And when did it become an acceptable risk for a patient to suffer any consequences of surgery or medical care? Where is the document that made the existence of any consent form possible? That's the one I'd like to see. I bet whoever drew it up made the doctors sign a waiver so the consent form didn't apply to the health care of the law partners who designed the agreement. Who created this blame-free medical system? Why is it *an acceptable risk* for me to die from an infection or bleeding out during surgery or merely lose a leg, get permanent nerve damage, or be paralyzed? I thought the whole purpose we're paying doctors is *not* to make mistakes. What if all jobs were like theirs? For example, professional baseball. Can you imagine a player saying this to an owner, "Before I agree to play for your club, sign this consent form that says I'm not required to get clutch hits with the bases loaded, and I'm not responsible for my fielding errors because those are acceptable risks in the game. After all, you can't blame me if I'm performing professionally to the best to my ability." I guess the larger question in this due-diligence issue is what type of consent form can I ask a physician to sign? "Here you go doc, before your work on me, this consent form states if you fail, you're required to return my fees, and if an investigation reveals you made an avoidable error that physically incapacitates me or causes my death, or if I or my estate are financially unable cover my future medical costs or sue you because you successfully lobbied to put caps on malpractice suits, this consent form before you, *absolves me or anyone who knows me* from being sued or charged with assault after we beat the shit out of you." What does the physician risk? I'll tell you one risk most doctors won't take: providing care for anyone without checking if their insurance covers the procedure.

Can you imagine what would happen if a patient entered an oncology exam or surgery, accompanied by their lawyer? The doctors would drop the patient's folder, tear off their stethoscope and run screaming from the room.

They live by litigation, we die from it.

AN HOUR LATER, I'M IN PRE-OP, WEARING A HOSPITAL GOWN, lying in a gurney while the nurse takes vital signs. My anxiety train jumps into balls-to-the-wall autopilot. It spins closer and closer to my head in a tightening circle as it winds around my one-track mind. Will there be an earthquake during surgery and the surgeon's scalpel will sever an artery? What about MERSA or SEPSIS or other hospital-born infections? Will the anesthesiologist bungle my injection and I'll never wake up? The brain is a smug, self-satisfied organ. I don't listen to my stomach when it has indigestion so why do I listen to my brain when it has anxiety? *Because it tells me to!* I decided not to bring up my fears because it might throw the surgeon or anesthesiologist off their game and cause them to make a mistake. It's like telling the pitcher in the fifth inning they have a no-hitter going. Some things you don't mess with.

My surgeon enters. I decide to open with my Democrat testicle joke.

"After the operation, I can officially say that—"

He interrupts me. Great, another tough room—and even worse, a bad straight man who ruined the set-up for my joke.

"I've performed hundreds of these operations," said my surgeon, Dr. Over Confident, but with a reassuring certainty that irritates instead of relaxes me. He wasn't comforting. Maybe I too defensive. The last time I heard a surgeon speak in a self-assured tone, Dad wound up dead. This surgeon could have performed millions of these operations but *this is my first one with him*. Confidence is how the *surgeon* gets through the operation not the patient. I wonder if doctors grasp how traumatic it is for the patient to wake up feeling carved out because a blade reached into them and extracted an organ? Part of you is actually flicked onto a scrap heap.

I suggest a possible prosthetic to replace the missing testicle.

"No," he snaps firmly. "You know why?"

"Because I have a screen in there from a hernia?"

"It's because of the scar tissue from it. We can put one in later, even two."

"I'm not going to go under again for another operation to put in false testicles, how about putting in a pair of fuzzy dice on the outside instead—you know, the ones you see hanging from rear-view mirrors in fifties cars?"

No response. Has a previous patient worked this room and stolen my lines?

"Do you have any more questions?"

"Can you use my port to administer the anesthetic?"

"We have to use an IV. It's the most effective method to administer anesthesia."

"Okay."

Dr. Over Confident exits. I thought, before he goes into surgery, he'll probably stop at Asgard to bitch about mortals to the other Gods.

The anesthesiologist inserts the dreaded IV in my left arm.

"I hate these needles," I glumly said, turning my face to the wall. "These needles make me feel like I'm in prison."

Dr. Quick, the anesthesiologist enters with a male assistant. He's in his thirties. A nice guy. Good eye contact. He went to school in San Diego.

I said, "I've been paddling out in the water to get in shape for this."

Dr. Quick said, "Between classes I'd run down and surf Black's on a longboard."

I'm thinking, I hope this guy caught the swell but made it back in time to the class on how to prevent complications that cause death from anesthesia.

I asked, "How long will the effects of sedation stay with me after the operation?"

Dr. Quick's assistant smirked and quipped, "A year from now at this same time you should be fine."

I laughed. *At last*, a funny guy who gets it! But I'm edgy. They give me a drug to relax me. I feel a little floaty. I lose my shoreline grip, go along with it, and drift out to the sloppy sea of me. Soon I'll be transferred to the operating room. Tears begin to flow. Will I open my eyes again?

The nurse notices my nervousness and gently said to me, "Are you okay, Fred?"

I nod, wipe the tears away and reply, "What can I tell you?" I add, "The only good thing is after the operation I'll never have to say, 'Three times is the charm.'"

"Oh," she softly spoke, sadness in her eyes. I expected a laugh, but I guess what I said was too true. The joke wasn't funny to her, but it was happening to me. I wasn't offended. But she was right, I guess.

"Yeah I know, too soon," I said, about the timing of the joke.

Before I had a bat and ball to play with. Soon I'll be down to a bat. It might improve my disposition — I'll be less *crotch*ety. I'll never do anything half cocked. My only guarantee: The guy who comes out of this is *definitely* going to be different than the one going in.

My sperm was down for the count.

MY PLUCK-AND-TUCK ORCHIECTOMY IS AN IN-AND-OUT PROCEDURE.
Years ago, when I first had surgery to remove my left testicle, I was in the hospital the night before and spent another two days there recovering from the operation. The incision was about three or four inches and looked like a vagina with staples in it. Not exactly a genital-like orifice a guy wants to see in his groin — even if I got horny and wanted to violate myself, I couldn't possibly reach it. This second time, they admit me into the hospital at 11:30 A.M. and four hours later, I'm

discharged and driven home percolating on percodans. I wonder if my health plan puts me in the 12-or-less-organs express checkout lane ("Hey, he only had one testicle, she has two breasts and an hysterectomy, he's first in line.") Besides being able to wear tighter pants, and confusing the hell out of the next tailor trying to find my inseam, what goes with a no-testicles look? I mulled over a few options to fill-in the storage gap in my testicle-evicted scrotum…

ALTERNATIVE USES FOR MY EMPTY NUT SACK

- Put a slit in the sack to hold stamps, car keys or tokens for tolls on the parkway.
- Tea cozy.
- Stuff it with fortunes like a cookie.
- Fill with malted Milk Balls.
- Be a surrogate for marsupials.
- Change purse.
- Maracas.
- Store license and registration.
- Wireless speakers that play "The Balls of Montezuma."
- Fill sack with steel balls so TSA has to inspect it at the airport.
- Use it to smuggle candy into movie theaters.
- Zip-lock seal to keep sandwiches fresh.
- Mulling wine spice bag.
- Install a clapper to turn on or turn off erections.
- Speed bag for hostile women to release out their job stress.
- Sachet of potpourri.
- Install false testicles that talk when you squeeze them.(The one on the left says,"Turn" and the right one say "Cough.").
- Speaker phone.
- Use ball bearings to create a dangling Newton's cradle.

I RELUCTANTLY LOOK IN THE MIRROR AT MY CARVED-UP PHYSIQUE. My naked body has been strip-mined and clearcut. I haven't been reduced to a sexual object — I'm a *reduced* sexual object. With my last testicle gone, it's like I have a crumbled candy wrapper between my legs. The incision is an inflamed slash of a three-inch smirk atop a small puffy inflamed mound above my crotch that flashes out an occasional sharp pain deep in the folds of my flesh. I look at the cut, it's like cancer attempted a larger bite out of me and missed. My pepper sprinkle of returning hair makes me look like a badly watered Chia pet. The slight lump above my collarbone where the medical port is implanted resembles a rivet (When I shower I still can't bring myself to touch it, I tamp it with a cloth.). The scars on my back from catheters are compounded by chemo-burn scars *inside* me. Tears ignited and burn my eyes. I think, man, what a journey. Who'd ever believe I had to unpack baggage to take this trip? The operation is behind me. So is my testicle. So is chemo. So are the catheters and urine bags. I'm wounded with character lines. The tears keep coming, trying to cleanse cancer from my field of vision so I could see whatever is coming at me again.

The next day, I get a phone. It was Dr. Over Confident. He identified himself by his first name not his title and said, "The testicle was in pretty bad shape. The good part is there is *no trace of cancer* on the testicle, which means there's an increased possibility that the tumor will only be scar tissue."

Well, there it is — or *was*.

"Thank you, I appreciate the call," I said, a little embarrassed. I realized Dr. Over Confident wasn't that bad a guy. *I had the wrong attitude.* So, factor in cancer, chemo, and a lost nut and grade me on a curve. But I unfairly misinterpreted his demeanor. That bothers me. Something else is wrong with my attitude, and I don't know what it is — yet.

Hours later in the middle of the night, I was jolted awake by a throb of pain where the surgeon cut above my groin to pluck the pulp of my testicle from the bloom of its sack. An adhesive sticky coating seals the rising welt of the curved slice. They had to remove my testicle because it was abnormal. Come on, I'm a guy. All testicles are abnormal! The loss carpets a stillness on me. My body is a silent landscape. I breathe over it. It's quiet — too quiet. I think of those scenes in Westerns movies where a frontier family is in their cabin and horrifyingly realize the bird calls they are hearing are really Indian signals and they're going to be slaughtered by Apaches. I've been scalped, for sure. The slight pain in my groin flares. It's less than I've felt before, like it's sinking and getting absorbed in the depths of healthy tissues.

It's been as real at it gets for how long? Endlessly, truly, madly, and deeply.

THE DAY AFTER MY UNCOSMETIC TESTICLE-REDUCTION SURGERY, I'M GREETED BY THE GUEST APPEARANCE OF FRED'S AMAZING TECHNICOLOR CROTCH. After most operations, blood goes to the lowest point in the body. In my case: the penis. Of course, if I was Fred-17 this wouldn't happen because that organ would be the *highest* point of my body. The blood rush made the shaft of my penis widen and turn purple. It looks like an eggplant. Some people have purple hearts. I have a purple hard-on. When I walk my penis actually bangs like a bell clapper against the sides of my legs. It makes me feel like a gorilla during mating season. And, to brag a little, it's the first time I have to use an overlapping golf grip to urinate. But being this well endowed doesn't last long, what's new? So much for low hanging fruit — or eggplant.

FOOD BOOMERANGS BACK TO ME. I'm was on my lunch break at a part-time job in a winery tasting room. I sat outside on a patio in a chair and took out a peach and bit into it. I felt the juice dribble down my mouth and onto my fingers. I stared at the rich and vibrant fruit surrounding the dark pit. I held a peach harvested from the world of light and water and earth. I was overcome by the taste. The compression of a vibrating high-amplitude wave built up inside me, then split in two, and rolled out toward my head and feet, completely overwhelming me. This G-force flavor scrunched my face. My lips quivered and the tears rolled again. Suddenly, a sensory bubble popped and stuck to my lips. I burst through a barrier and looked at the trees, felt the breeze. Everything was within reach. I was back in the world with a peach.

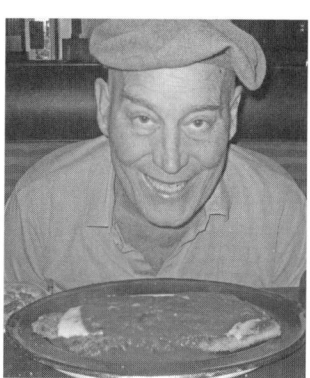
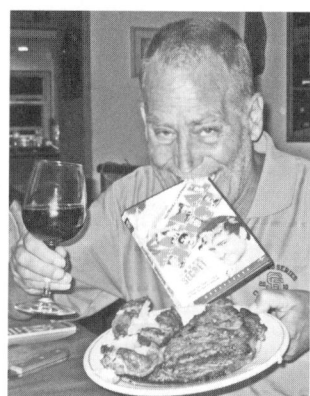

Dream of your hunger for comfort foods. It will nourish a belief you'll return to the flavor of you. Never underestimate the power of wine and a rib-eye, a cheeseburger, veal Parmesan, or a Sorrento's Sub from Freehold, New Jersey!

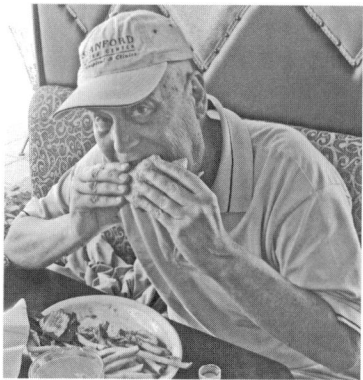
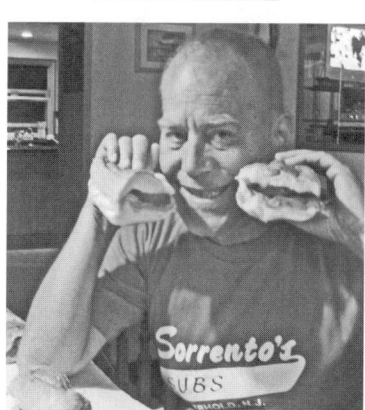

I CAN'T ABANDON MY LITTLE CACTUS BUDDY. For weeks, its dried stem with withered leaves was a whittled stick in the center of a soggy dirt-filled Popeye Spinach can. One day, I was tempted to chuck the can into the woods. I didn't want to be reminded he was dead. Instead, I kept watering my buddy. After a few days, I noticed the water was disappearing. Maybe it was merely evaporating, but I hoped the plant, even though it looked so dead, had a probing root of life still tingling in the soil. After all, he was a cactus! They're used to hard times in dryness. I rescued him at the start of my treatment, nurtured him along, then an uninvited circumstance uprooted him. I could relate. I tried to dismiss what happened to the cactus. After all, it wasn't a "he." It was just a plant. But I couldn't get past it. I kept watering and watering.

A week later, the cactus still looked as dead as could be. But I wasn't giving up on the little guy. My life couldn't spare any time for the inevitable.

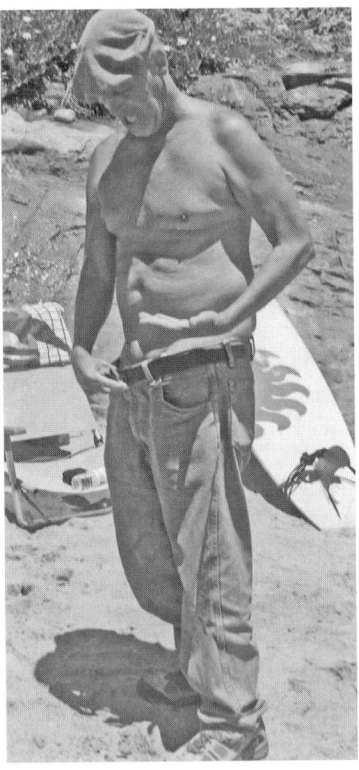

Hello, hello, is there anybody in there?
That's funny, I never heard an echo down there before.

HANGING NONE

My sex drive pulls into the urologist's service station for a premium-grade testosterone fill-up. Without testicles and no sperm, I'm running on fumes. My sperm-count gauge reads 5 in a tank that holds the 300-plus. What kind of fuel upgrade should I go with? Leaded or unleaded? Diesel? *Ball*-samic vinegar? Maybe there's an alternative way I can go electric — then again, where would I have to plug the recharger? There are parts of my body I don't want to attach jumper cables to! Besides, my crotch won't need a smog check because I don't have any emissions. It's odd to know I'll always be Jonesing for a testosterone fix for the rest of my life — women who have gone through menopause don't consider my hormonal dependence as a big deal, which reveals more about how people who *don't have* testosterone think. In a way, I feel like my penis has been reduced to a placeholder. It's like being stuck between gears. The only way normally-equipped males experience any lack of testosterone is holding their girlfriend or wife's purse while she tries on an outfit in the women's dressing room of a clothing store, or suppressing a laugh when she cries during a chick flick.

There are 4 ways to fill-up at the testosterone pump: **1.**) A testosterone gel to rub on your upper arms. If have pets, wash your hands after you apply it — unless you want your dog or cat to buy a 4-wheel drive truck, drink too much Jagermeister and get into bar fights. **2.**) Give yourself an under-the-skin shot every couple weeks. No, not there! Any other place — unless you're really weird. **3.**) Wear a patch on your arm 24-7. That's stupid. Who wants to wear a sperm merit badge? **4.**) Get a tiny incision in your butt cheek and have pellets of testosterone inserted into its slit and stitched in place, which keeps your hang-time going for three to four months. I didn't want to give myself a needle or wear a patch. I was told the gel is just as effective as having testosterone inserted, but I decided to get pellets implanted in my hip because I've always believed penetration was more manly. I've grown attached to propulsion.

Dr. Michael Eisenberg, my urologist, is a courteous, dark-haired, quietly intense guy. He looks like a cross between a *Star Trek* crew member and a young

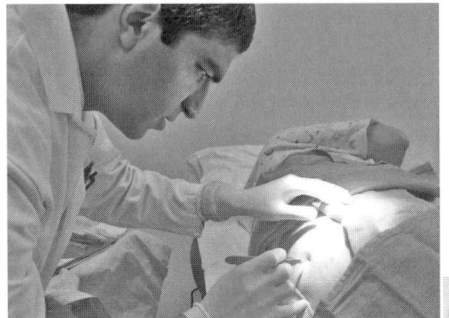

Dr.. Michael Eisenberg inserts tiny pellets of testosterone into me. He's turned my butt into a Pez dispenser. Nice Urologist Game Face too!.

Israeli Mossad agent in an espionage movie. I wonder if it's proper to ask if he's an absolute whiz in urology, but I guess it's like asking a proctologist if he's getting *behind* in his work. I always restrain myself from making obvious jokes about people's professions or last names — unless they're a harpist, or I don't like the person and want to piss them off, or they're a person I don't like who is also a harpist and I *really* want to piss them off. I guess I have harpist issues – good.

"Your testosterone levels are very low," said Dr. Eisenberg, who sits down and in a solemn tone asks, "So how have you been feeling?"

"Outside of the menstrual cramps, fine. I've also noticed I've been crying watching daytime TV talks shows about relationships and have a desire to go clothes shopping with my wife. And I may have an ovarian cyst."

It's half a tough room. There's a student assistant who laughs. Dr. Eisenberg just stares at me, not sure how to react. Understandable.

"Come on, if I want to feel nostalgic I have to ask you to turn and cough," I said. "Those jokes are funny. I was working on those lines last week!"

"When is the last time you had an erection?"

"Not since chemo," I replied, but I was tempted to say, "When I first saw your deep brown eyes enter this room." I decided not to go there. Wise move, huh?

A young Filipino nurse enters the room. She is stocky, wide-eyed, and smiles.

"Right now all I am is a vibrator with legs," I said then add the tag line, "You're looking at the most attractive lesbian from Santa Cruz." The student assistant laughs. The Filipino nurse stares. I'm surprised she didn't laugh. "I should be very popular with lesbians. I look like a guy and have none of that messy aftertaste." The assistant laughs. But still no reaction from the Filipino nurse. I wonder about it, but I guess her reaction makes more sense than a guy who is no longer a stand-up comedian, doesn't have testicles and tells self-deprecating dick jokes to his urologist.

A few other students enter the room to watch the procedure, all guys. This is the main priapic event. Dr. Eisenberg is going to administer the testosterone. He elaborates on why testosterone is important, "Testosterone you need for muscles and bones, affects your heart, sex drive —"

"How do you know if a guy hasn't been given *enough* testosterone?"

"They get fatigued and have less energy."

"Then how do you know when a guy has *too much* testosterone?"

Dr. Eisenberg thought a moment then said, "The wives complain."

"About what? The sex?"

"No, they complain the guy *argues* too much."

I laugh then reply, "Wait, a guy's been emasculated, actually lost his balls and his warhead is deactivated and he's *not quiet enough*?" He smiled. "I think wives confuse arguing with *refusing to obey*. After all, it's so rare for married couples to argue. But if a woman argues it's okay because as you know it's our fault we don't understand them. Wait, if guys have too much testosterone they become argumentative, defensive and don't listen. I always thought that's what estrogen does to women."

Dr. Eisenberg smirks. I'm clearly not your typical testicle-challenged castrato. It was go time.

I wondered if testosterone pellets were shaped like hand grenades or maybe replicas of the tiny plastic army soldiers I played with as a kid. With each soldier in a different combat position. What can I say? I think of testosterone as an armed force pointing a rifle or wielding some kind of firearm. Let's face it: it's ammo. I get reloaded every four months or my rifle jams.

"What does the testosterone look like?" I ask.

Dr. Eisenberg shows me these tiny square pellets. They look like teensy Chiclets. I lie on my side. He numbs my hip. Makes a small incision and slides the pellets one by one into the opening.

I turn and say, "You know, you're turning my ass into a Pez Dispenser."

All the students bend over and laugh. The Filipino nurse stares and blinks.

I shrug and say, "What else do you want me to say? There's nothing I can do about this." I laugh. "I'm cracking myself up." I turn to the wall. I stop laughing. He inserts more pellets. I lower my voice, "The toughest part coming here was passing the children's hospital."

"You mean the traffic?" he says.

"No, just knowing children are suffering like I suffered," I softly croak, my voice cracking. "It just tears me apart."

After they finish up, I'm alone with the Filipino nurse who never laughed.

"I'm sorry I didn't laugh," she said. "I don't find jokes funny. Sometimes I laugh when people laugh after they tell them so I don't hurt their feelings."

"Let me try one."

"Okay, but I won't laugh."

"A salesman has a cold and a sore throat. He knocks on a door, a woman answers. The salesman says (*I lower my voice to a whisper.*): 'Is your husband home?' She replies (*I lower my voice to a female whisper.*): 'No, come on in.'" The nurse smiles, wide-eyed, blinking at me like a koi fish. I try another one. "A duck goes into a pharmacy and asks for a condom. The druggist says, 'Do you want me to put that on your bill?' The bird replies, 'What *kind* of duck to you think I am?'" Again she goes into full-on koi. "Okay, a salesman knocks on a door. A teenager answers. He's in his underwear, smoking dope, drinking scotch and rap music is playing. Salesman says, 'Are your parents home?' Kid exhales smoke from a bong and says, 'What the fuck *do you think?*'" Again she goes koi. I shake my head. "I got nothing." I crack up and say, "You don't laugh at jokes — that's funny."*

She seemed embarrassed and apologetically says, "I told you."

"It's okay," I reply. "You're a very nice lady. That's all that matters." I added with a smile, "The joke's on me, really."

If you think about my situation, what's really so funny? Well, funny's *something I have to be*. They say humor is a defense mechanism. Not if you use it right.

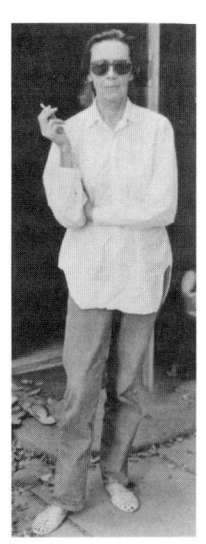

There are people in your life who are gone, but their influence shaped your character. If you've lived a good life, when you're ill, their voices will come to save you.

I FOUND ANOTHER SEED OF ME TO GROW BACK: two lovers flee a gigantic ferocious rose that's violently bursting out the doors and windows of their country cottage. That's the painting Jean made that came back to me after I finished Chekhov's short story, *The Black Monk*. I hadn't thought about Jean Jackson in a long time. But cancer brings people back to you. She was an artist. A successful one too. She was born in New York in 1907. Studied at the Academie

Julien in Paris and the Art Students League in New York. Her fantasy paintings of animals, children and apparitions had been exhibited in New York since the 1940's, at the Iolas Gallery, the Maynard Walker Gallery and the Betty Parsons Gallery, and were bought by prominent collectors, among them Paul Mellon and the Metropolitan Museum of Art. In Chekhov's *The Black Monk*, the main character Kovin tells the legend about a monk dressed in black, who wandered in the desert 1,000 years ago and set off a series of mirages. His image is seen walking in different countries all over the world. This monk returns to Earth and reappears to men. The monk visits Kovin, who has the potential talent to become a great artist. The monk says, "I exists in your imagination, and your imagination is part of nature, so I exist in nature... If you want to be healthy and normal go to the common herd." Kovin settles for economic security and doesn't pursue the path of his talent, and years later, laments, "I was interesting and original. Now I have become more sensible and stolid, but I am just like everyone else: I am — mediocrity." Kovin continues to talk to the monk no one sees but him. People think he's insane. His obsession with the loss of his talent destroys his marriage and the lives of others. Kovin realizes this obsession has ruined him, he bewails the life he missed, his ruined marriage, and dies. At the tale's end, the Black Monk concludes Kovin died because "his frail human body had lost its balance and could no longer serve as the moral garb of genius."

I met Jean through a friend in Connecticut. She was in her seventies. A statuesque wisp of a woman. My Mom met her and said, "She must have been a beauty when she was younger." I was in my twenties. Jean took a benevolent and nurturing proprietary interest in me because I read books and aspired to be a writer. She showed me a scrapbook with articles about her. There was a photo of Jean with Salvador Dali. There was also a copy an early painting of a lovers fleeing in horror from a monstrous rose ("I thought it was funny, nobody else did," she said). Jean twisted animation into anything. One time I opened a novel she had in her house and found an elm leaf she used for a bookmark — with a few deft black brush strokes she painted the leaf so it looked like a fish. She told me about her life as an artist, fashion model for *Vogue* and how she was angry she missed her chance to fuck Jack Kerouac ("I almost had him!"). Anytime she spotted a chaotic creative spark Jean's eyes widened, she'd press her lips, take a long draw on a cigarette and as its spark glowed she made an mmm-sound of purring pleasure and said, "Marvelous."

There were many pieces of advice Jean gave me: "Every unattractive woman knows a pretty one... There's an interesting reason why someone is boring... A rich person in a group will somehow take everyone's money. They're like magnets... All men have one particular dish they're good at making... An actor is only happy when they're someone else." I remember giving her a novel, and when I saw her later, she said, "I read a few pages and stopped. I'm nearing the end of my life and need inspiration. And this book is just clever. And anyone can be clever. You can take the dullest knife and sharpen it."

Jean believed in reincarnation. She said, "I'm trying to master watercolor to take that skill into the next life." The day she was moving away with her husband to Hayesville, South Carolina. I knew I'd never see her again. She tried to compensate for the spreading gap between us by filling it with a variety of books and a drawing she did for my birthday. The day before she died, she said to her husband, "I got it. Watercoloring. I've finally got it!" He found her lying in the garden, claw marks from her fingernails in the dirt by her hands. *The New York Times* ran her obituary.

Before Jean left, I told her I decided to pursue stand-up comedy. Her eyes widened as she inhaled her cigarette. One more happy fool marching to the madness parade. Jean's smile and widening eyes and mmm-purr brush strokes basted away the lure of clever. If I settled for clever, instead of chucking it all and going to California, I'd have remained a journalist in Connecticut, and after ten years of cynicism, probably wound up at a public relations gig in New York City, then gotten married, had a kid, moved to Fairfield County or a Jersey suburb, commuted on a train to The City, spent my weekends at a racquetball spa or a country club and end up with a bad back and bum knees — and cancer. Or instead of going the corporate route, stuck to journalism for thirty years only to have a new owner "restructure" the newspaper, and get laid off without benefits or severance, and get cancer. Okay, Fred-57 was broke, in debt, and had cancer, but what if I ended up this same way and was still back East, would I have regretted my choice? I think so, because I have no regrets now. If I never lit out for California, the infusion of the life I didn't live would have finished me. I'd have ended up as a first-draft character in an unpublished John Cheever short story riding the Westport-New York commuter train in the bar car. I remembered those stolid men. Middle-aged guys who boasted about their professional accomplishments as they pounded down drink after drink and made viper-like observations about corporate politics and trumpet their lifestyle or income. But in the middle of their fourth vodka or fifth-scotch snort, "It's all bullshit." My young, vainly withdrawn, judgmental and self-conscious mind assessed them but never factored myself in any equation because I was in denial my career was descending in their direction. Whatever they extinguished didn't define what I could still do with my life. I manned up. I faced my responsibilities and ran away from them.

In comedy I avoided clever and *went towards feel*. The cleverest comics were the harshest guys. They had the greatest contempt for the audience. They were superb at manipulating the crowd, calculating jokes, and creating a false engaging image of themselves. This gave these comics an deeper intense disdain for their fans, because the character on the stage wasn't the person the audience loved. The joke was really on them: in the end the laughs and love they craved were for someone else. And those comics' egos were more self-centered and driven then any CEO. They were ambitious and cunningly obsequious and usually succeeded in a sitcom for a few years, then were forgotten, and replaced by another younger flavor. After that, if they didn't become game-show hosts, they mutated into the most bitter people in show business: comics who became comedy writers. Why? *Because they gave up performing.* They'd let some other talent harvest their best pulp — pulp that should have been the fruit of their own bits and pieces. If you polish someone else's star you can't be the sheriff in your own town. And dammit, when the bad guy is shooting up the place, I wanted to be the man to take him down. These writers had incisive, cutting, dark and satiric-cleaver minds. It's a seductive and cruel intelligence. Their lines burns like napalm down to the bone and left nothing for anyone else. I thought it was amusing most comics became funny because a bully hurt their feelings, or from some personal wound, but here they were using funny the same way a bully used his muscles to hurt weaker people and wound others. They rarely laughed unless they were burned by the poker of brutally pointed observation about their ego or talent from the dissecting perspective of another person just like them. I'd see these well-paid writers drinking hard liquor at the comedy club bar, seething as the comic on stage gets laughs. They glare at the comic and spit out, "He never does my lines right." And I wanted to say, "The reason isn't because he's not saying them correctly, the reason is: *you're not saying them.*" But sometimes you can become a person you don't like when you fight and compete to do what you do best. At times, I was guilty of that sin too, and I regret it.

Jean showed me we all possess a quirky but yet undefined uniqueness it's our choice to develop, it could be for anything, accounting, raising a family, knitting, pottery, or whatever. The purest core of us is an idiosyncratic fanfare that announces our presence to a room. It's the pilot light that goes out when your shrunken body is lying in state without you in it. Some don't want to make the sacrifice and their lava becomes a dry ocean bed and their caramelized dreams fossilize in it. If your passion becomes your hobby, you've embalmed yourself. I didn't want to end up wearing the dented halo of a dimly glowing life. I never dimmed my pilot light with cleverness. Maybe that's why no one could ever convince me I was less than what I desired to be. You don't have to work with a net if you can fly. The hardest thing in life is to be yourself. It takes a long time to drill down and tap into the spring of the natural resource of *your voice*. Its tight bud unconsciously bursts out. It's what's inside you that you never see coming. I'd unexpectedly taste it on the stage, writing, improvising on the radio, pelting a pure shot in golf, pulling an instinctive move surfing an unpredictable wave. When your in the zone of your locked-in automatic pilot light, everyone around you knows you're on fire because you look so consumed. That's the angry flame where I stoked my life and forged its spirit into an blistering orange-glow and dove off the high-dive into the tumor's core, held the breath of all of me until I touched The Big C's bottom and incinerated and evaporated its malignancy into a moist and burbling and splashing and spraying and steaming hiss. What can I say? It worked for me.

Marvelous, right Jean?

SURVIVING CANCER DOESN'T MEAN YOUR LIFE ENDS. You retain the spirit that got you through treatment but you still have to make a living and deal with middle-management people who produce nothing. They're only good at one thing: keeping their jobs *while everyone else is doing their job*. Through office politicking they maneuver themselves atop a pile of more talented coworkers, which enables these lessers to reach the low hanging fruit from the branches of their limited ambition. They thrive in a system to set you up to fail or throw you under the bus. You can be a perfectly decent person and they will come after you. If they ask for your opinion at work, and you give it, they decide you're argumentative and not a team player. They do everything they can to get in your way. You can't defeat them in their cubicle hive. They're better at lying than you are at finding out the truth. They are the people you have to be *paid* to get along with at work, but who *don't feel* they have to get along with you. And if you dare point out that contradiction in their team-building philosophy, they'll make your life miserable, and devise a way to eventually get you fired. They are only concerned about what's between them and their food dish. Their only goal? Getting a bigger food dish. These flat-affect people have unreflecting eyes (A cold stove doesn't have a pilot light.). They're cancer's role models. *And they're exactly like cancer because they can only exist and thrive in a system but are unable to live outside of it.* Their personal lives are train wrecks. Their ambition turns against them and they don't even realize it. That's why they live for work and make everyone else's jobs a living hell. They enjoy seeing how their misery tastes in the mouths of others. They dread unbearable stretches of free time. They'd rather be at work! Why? Because in their solitude they have nothing to offer even to themselves. And the reason? These people compartmentalize their personal life and working relationships to benefit themselves. And deny those separate-but-equal compartments are rooms in a house they built on a false foundation for their comfort. This Mystery House of Them is never completed or available for parties. They keep frantically building addition after addition until all this disassociation expands and collapses of its own weight, and crumbles about them and they find themselves standing in the rubble and discover no one is there for them. They misinterpret their self-imposed demolishment as proof no one in life cares about anybody but themselves. When these people become ill, or get lonely, they have no choice but to depend on the kindness of *complete* strangers who professionally care for them out of a sense of duty not love "because it's the right thing to do."

MY PET SCAN IS TOMORROW. They'll shoot glucose into me. Cancer loves glucose. It digs sugar rushes because it never needs long-term energy to go the distance. If glucose glows in the tumor's interred remains, The Big C's heartless body is still beating within me. But, if there is only darkness, my light is born.

For good luck, I returned to Pleasure Point to give a nod to what inspired and gave me endurance: my surf spot. This place is the closest I come to going inside a church and *liking it*. There's a swell. A horde of clueless fake-cool people out in the water. I look between the crowd to see my ocean — it was still there.

Odwallah Ken came by on an old Schwinn bike to check out the surf. He's called Odwallah Ken because he works for Odwallah juice drinks. That's how surfers name people. If you're a fireman, you're Fireman Jim. Like barbecue? Barbecue Bob. Your surf break is near 38th street? You surfed 38th. Or near an old sewer pipe? Sewers. Surfers never have to develop a vocabulary, instead of saying things like "He worked assiduously to achieve a penultimate triumph in his field," a surfer says, "The bro is hella wicked sick at his bomb job."

When I was in chemo land, Ken went out of his way to give me protein drinks.

"I got it earlier this morning when no one was on it," said Ken, looking at the waves, smiling. "Scored." He paused. "I haven't seen you in awhile."

"I've been coming down on flat days just to paddle," I said.

A stern-faced pudgy short woman in a wetsuit, wielding a pointed surfboard like a shield, defiantly strutted by us as if she was a warrior ready to do battle.

"Check that out," I said, imitating her macho strut and angry body language. "If that's the way she's going into the water, I hate to see what she's like out there." I paused. "I don't have people like that in my personal life. So why would I want to be around them doing what I love to do?"

"Yeah, they're a lot of them," said Kenny. He nodded at the shorebreak to a middle-aged, short, pot-bellied surfer. The guy was getting out of the ocean, flipping off someone in the surf, grumbling to himself. "Look who's coming in." The guy was a sour, foul-mouthed surfer in the water, who intimidated people so he could get more waves. I had gotten into it with him many times.

"I don't even call that guy by his name, he's just a 'Hey, hi' to me," I replied. "Why give him an identity?" I smiled. "Not that I have an opinion."

"If you stay here, you'll hear a him complain about everyone and everything."

I tensed up. I had no room for the bitter vaporings of a self-centered moron. Stay where love remains, I thought. Stay where love remains.

"I'll pass," I said, leaving. "You know I have to fight the cancer that still might be inside me." I nodded in the direction of the approaching surfer. "I don't want to see the cancer cells *outside* of my body." I smiled. "The way I look at people like him is when I close my eyes he's gone, when he closes his eyes, he's still there. He's his own problem. I don't want him to be mine, anymore."

Kenny cracks up and said, "Can't imagine what you're going through, I figured the best I could do was help."

"You have helped me, thank you for those juices," I said. "The ocean and your kindness are what I want to leave here with and take with me tomorrow. All I can do is bring what I love with me into the hospital. That's all I can do. Bring the good to push back the darkness. That's why I *had to* come here. It's why I always come here. I want to be here for good."

When I return home, I check my little cactus. I happily discover a tightly wound green bud atop the plant's brown stalk. *He's alive!* My buddy pulled through. The shape of his teeny coiled greenness spreads out a warmth in me that ascends like a puck from a mallet blow to a pivot and soars up my wired spine and rings the bell atop the Feat-Of-Strength carnival game's tower in my head. Clang! My cactus was back with me again!

I choke heavily breaths out, "Eh, eh, eh, eh."

Each "eh" scrunches my face tighter and tighter. My lips pucker. Tears flow. A feeling of the endlessly unwinding of everything hits me. The knot of anxiety is a straight piece of string without a motive. The cactus and I swing from it.

It's a promising sign.

It was nice to know something outside of me is growing again.

In the middle of the night before my pet scan, a familiar intruder enters our bedroom...

"Fred! Fred! Fred!" Laurie shrieks in fear, bolting upright in bed.

"What?" I asked, alarmed.

"I had this dream, this big hairy creature like the one in *Star Wars*."

"Chewbacka?"

"Yes, he was on our bed, in a white jumpsuit, jumping up and down."

"It's okay, it's okay."

I knew who Chewbacka was. He was Death using his all-access pass. During chemo, I was accustomed to Mr. D, his empty darkness was part of the decor. When I first had testicular cancer, we head-butted. He'd always pop up uninvited with his eternal sense of entitlement. Mr. D's 3 a.m. appearance doesn't perturb me. I'm accustomed to his moods. He can jump on this bed all night. Go right ahead, jump all you want. You're rocking me to sleep. I appreciate it. It's helping. I'm going to live to get up early tomorrow morning. And then some.

Time to launch my pet offensive on the "heterogeneously enhancing mass located adjacent to the iliacus muscle." I'm escorted to a 65-degree room that's housing yet another scanner that resembles a combination gigantic front-loading washing machine and spaced-aged pizza oven. Am I going to be dry cleaned or flipped on a spatula? A technician places my upraised arms into a pillowcase above my head to prevent me from moving. I'm strapped down to a flat table. I'm wrapped in blankets. I look like a body for a burial at sea. I'm told the scan will take 30–40 minutes. The table retracts into the antiseptic futuristic-looking vacuum tube. I hear the machine's flying-saucer-like whirring. Beams flash. I've become a chunk of pulsating red meat slapped on a slide, getting stripped, filleted and freeze framed. I felt like I was looking up through the opposite end of a microscope into the giant eye of a value judgment.

Within the narrow cylinder, a fuzzy relapse into panic settles upon my body like a flock of crows feeding on me as if I'm clinical road kill. Have I been under the illusion of survival this whole time? Is my resolve just a primer coat of denial trying to paint out my death date? Could I go through chemo again? Yes. Could I live through a complex operation to remove the tumor from an artery? Wait, this isn't me thinking! The Big C is throwing its voice inside me. *Don't let It in.*

I cry and harshly whisper, "You're not there, you're not there."

My soul is arcing and stretching.

As the spin-cycle of imaging swirls around me, tears come. They stream and make my cheeks itch. My arms are restrained in a pillowcase. I can't wipe the tears off. Nowhere to go. I'm stuck here for thirty minutes. I imagine I'm in a time tunnel. I flashback a few years to Dad's phone call from Connecticut.

"Fred, I have cancer in my colon," whimpered Dad. "I found out today. The doctor's are going to operated this coming Friday."

"I'll be there."

"It's a simple surgery. You don't have to come all the way out here for that."

"Hey, I only have *one* Dad."

There was a long silence at the end of the line. It was what Dad wanted to hear.

"That's right," he softly said. "You only have one."

"I'm leaving tomorrow."

Before Dad went into surgery, he was sitting up in a gurney, smiling, beaming and looking at me. There was admiration in his eyes. I felt what he was thinking: "My son gave up everything to be here. He'd risk his job. He'd lose money. No matter what, my son's Number One Priority and The Most Important Thing In The World is to be *here* for me." I believe a son becomes a man when he's there for his father. It was the proudest achievement of my life.

During visiting hours for the one-hundred-plus days Dad was in ICU, he was rarely alone. Cindy often held vigil. She played the drama card, big time. She gave the impression to nurses she was The *Only One In The Family* making an enormous personal sacrifice. A nurse said to me, "I admire your sister, she told her boss that he could fire her if he wanted but she was going to take care of her father. She put her life on hold for her dad." I said nothing. Cindy didn't have a job or a boss! She made and sold jewelry at arts-and-craft shows, and purchased items at estate sales she placed in consignment areas of antique stores. She was mainly supported by her boyfriend, who was a nice guy. She always exaggerated her importance, and became nasty if you challenged her exaggerated stories. *What happened to the sweetness in her I grew up with?* My brother came to the hospital after a carpeting job. *Why did he grow up to steal from Dad?* Stephanie spent most of the time passed out drunk in her room — she blamed her medication or a cold. Not once did I see her apologize to Dad. Why was I thinking about this now? Especially here! I received an answer that shamed me. My parents were talking to me, so I let the memory play out. The day before Dad died, Stephanie was by his bed. He ruefully gazed at her with a glazed and deep concern emanating from the center of a glistening yearning in his eyes. Dad didn't see a 52-year old alcoholic. He saw his lost little girl. What was going to become of his lost little girl? Dad's concern for Stephanie was greater than his disappointment in her. How it must have pained him. How his love for her made him blame himself instead of her. I realized that's how Mom and Dad viewed all of us. No matter what age we were, they only saw our best and promising qualities they hoped their love formed in us so we'd triumph over their shortcomings as well as our own and attain a better life. And my shortcoming is my inability to see my brother and sisters through my parents' eyes. As I was getting scanned, I let Mom and Dad's love in. It lasered away the cataracts formed by the pain, grief, resentment and financial stress my seemingly impervious siblings indifferently inflicted upon me. Just as my parents' love accused themselves instead of casting blame, I had see through my own disappointments and believe the love of Mom and Dad would redeem our family. My parents sacrificed so I could be a better man. If I kept my wounds open, I'd be as bad as people who spend their whole lives bitterly cooking meals on the dark side of overdone. And worse, I would have grown up short of my parents' dreams for me. I'd be a failure. I decided not to hold anything against my brother or sisters. My new goal was to be Bigger Than Me. I couldn't erase the financial costs they burdened me with on The Blackboard of My Life. So, I threw the slate away. It skipped off the surface of the past and sunk. I decided to call my brother and sisters once in awhile, and send them presents on the holidays and birthdays, and never bring up how they treated me in probate. I'd forgive, but I'd never depend on them to do the right thing or ever lend them money!

A recast Fred-57 was pulled out of the cylinder by the technician. I didn't ask her anything. She wasn't allowed to tell me the scan's outcome, anyway.

"I was told the results of my scan are STAT, and I should hear from the doctor today," I said.

"Yes, in a couple hours," she replied.

I didn't make eye contact with the technician. If she had pity in her eyes, I would be able to tell if she's bummed because her dog got hit by a car, or my PET scan had tumors lighting up all my organs like a morbid Christmas tree.

> **Stat:** A medical abbreviation for urgent or rush. From the Latin word statum, meaning 'immediately.'

THE RESULTS OF MY PET SCAN ARE STAT. But I don't immediately hear from anyone. I expected this — but I bet, if I was a fellow oncologist or related to my oncologist I'd get my scan results *faster* than STAT.

I called the Stanford Cancer Center for the results. I'm on hold and hear horrendous classical music with hard shrieking violins like the *Pyscho* soundtrack where Norman Bates deftly hacks up Janet Leigh in the motel shower.

A woman came back on the line, "Yes, Stanford Cancer Center."

"You need to change that music. It sounds like someone is being murdered."

"Yes, we've had complaints and we're—"

"When I hear it I think I've called Stanford Cancer Center and Funeral Home." She cracks up.

"I had a PET scan this morning. My oncologist was going to call me with the results in a couple of hours. It's pretty important. The test results will tell me if cancer is dead in my body, or I have to go through chemo again or a major operation. I'd kinda like to know the answer so it's easier for me to sleep tonight."

I hear rapid typing on a computer keyboard on her end, it sounds like a cat eating dry food from a bowl. The woman said my request is listed as STAT and she has sent it to the oncologist office. I thank her, hang up and wait.

No one called.

I was so exhausted steeling myself against the day's stress, I went to bed early and solidly slept through the night. In the morning, I called again. I was told I'd have my results by 3 P.M. Until then, everything was dead time.

THE JURY HAS REACHED A VERDICT. The phone rings at 3 P.M. Is it a death sentence for cancer or me? The oncologist's nurse gives me the PET scan results:

> **Impression**: 1. When compared to the prior exam, there has been a moderate decrease in size and FDG activity of hypermetabolic right external iliac nodal conglomerate. 2. No evidence of distant metastases.

And what does that mean? Here's the Oncological-to-English translation:

> **CANCER IS DEAD.**

"So you're telling me there's no glow in my pelvic area," I gulp, my voice cracking and tears flowing. I press my lips tightly together, trying to compose myself.

"Yes."

I choked out, "No glow or sign of cancer anywhere else?"

"No."

My entire body crumbles and I moan. Words catch in my mouth as I struggle to say, "So, I guess I'm going to open a nice bottle of wine tonight."

"You have something to celebrate."

My face clenches and I barely blurt out, "Thank you."

I call Laurie and say, "There is no cancer in me. It's dead."

She gasped and cried, "That's just so wonderful. I love you."
"Love you too. They say no glow so I'm a go."
"Well, I'm stopping and getting a rib-eye for someone," she said, hanging up.
"I made it," I said, clicking off my cell phone. I softly do an mmm-groan-moan gasp of gratitude. "I'm back." Tears warm my eyelids. I wetly sniff and sigh, hang my head and weakly warble to The Great Unknown, "Thank you."

I'm laughing as humbling tears of victorious struggle roll out and tickle me. I reach forward to dance with the future to the beat of a tune I can make out just over the horizon. I see new dawns with wearied but refreshed eyes. I'm released into my next life, but still can't cast off my coat of arms. I refuse drop my guard. I mistakenly thought this was a strength. It was a side effect — caused by me.

My victory dinner is a barbecued rib-eye steak, baked potato, a shrimp salad and a 10-year old Beauregard Vineyards Cabernet. I excitedly posted pictures of my celebratory meal on *Facebook*. You'd think I'd get encouragement but a woman wrote this comment:

> Fred, you spent months healing by poisoning your body with chemo. It poisoned the cancer out of you. So in a way, you did not heal, the chemo just killed the cancer. The foods you are choosing cause cancer. Red meat and dairy have been scientifically proven to cause cancer. Try eating foods that help your body to recover. Over time you will repoison yourself. Drink fruit smoothies. Eat apples, broccoli, healthy things like that. I'm happy that you are better, but it's a shame you do not choose to heal yourself.

As Dad used to say, "Another country heard from." Who can argue with protein and eating healthy? These Bunched-Greener vegan hug false gods of organic rice, wheat grass, and yeast. These yoga-breathing dragons are zealously reassured by the conviction their wholesome soy-powdered menu makes them invulnerable to cancer because their flaxseed-oil lubricated bodies have a low pH levels or some stupid mineral metabolic balancing act. Many people who ate healthy died from The Big C, such as Adele Davis, Linda McCartney, and others who are rich enough to afford a steady diet of organic foods. Hey, no one is safe! One sure symptom the protein-deprived brains of health-food nuts are in a truly heightened vegetative state is their mindset that instead of radiation or chemo, I should have undergone a holistic regimen to cure myself. I guess you undergo their prescribed cancer treatments of these self-appointed oncologists at the Bob Marley Memorial Hospital or The Steve Jobs Herbal Infusion Juice Bar. Cancer isn't afraid of vegetables. However, cancer might fear broccoli, which I suspect is a major chemo ingredient.

A Title Match at The Infusion Grand Arena
THE CHEMO KID
vs
THE BIG C
The Showdown of a Lifetime!

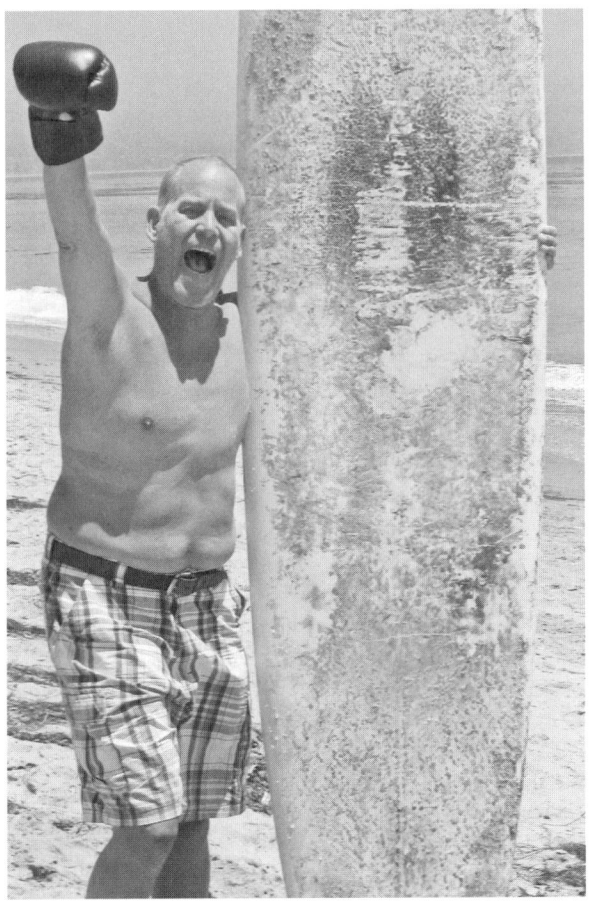

Round Four MY TOWER OF POWER IS GONE FROM MY CORNER. I'm not wearing a hospital robe or testicles. I'm in boxing trunks. My hair is growing back. I'm hungry and sharply home my focus on the inarticulate mass that did this to me: The Big C. He's sitting on a stool, thin and frail as a chemo patient. His tumor heart has completely dissolved inside him, turning his once transparent body a morbid gray. His muscles are no longer rippling and flowing, they've been replaced by stacks of disorganized binding and hardening crystals that are cracking sliver linings in his flesh and oozing out of his body. His figure is slowly congealing into a jelled blob.

The ringside commentator says, "The Chemo Kid's vital signs are: Blood Pressure 143/97. Pulse: 65. Temperature: 97.2. Respiration 18. Weight 206 LB. 2.1 OZ. You have to admire The Chemo Kid for withstanding such an unbelievable Infusion onslaught and coming back. What an incredible turnaround. The Big C is falling apart. This crowd is on its feet in a frenzy."

The bell clangs. I've finished chemo, now I finish him.

I bounce in the center of the ring, waiting for The Big C. With each step he takes, his body trails a rising cloud of dying cancer cells. He can't raise his gloves to defend himself. I'll show him the same mercy, he so graciously gave me.

"The Chemo Kid unleashes a brutal flurry of hooks, jabs, right and left crosses. Combination, combination, combination! Jab, jab, jab! Letting it all loose. It's relentless! The Chemo Kid is multiplying and dividing punches faster than The Big C can metastasize any kind of defense or attack. Body, head! Oh, what a shot! The Big C's in trouble, big trouble. The champ's backed into the corner."

"This is for taking my left nut," I shout landing a right to the Big C's head.

"Bingo!" said the commentator. "The Kid throws a jab to champ."

"This is for taking my right nut," I shout, slamming the other side of his temple, mashing it

The shared souls of spectators roar.

"Oh, boom!" cries the commentator. "A left cross lands The Big C on the ropes."

"And this — this is for killing my Mom!" I shout and ferociously throw a left hook, and follow it up with a right cross pounding into The Big C's midsection. "That's for killing my Dad!"

The commentator exclaims, "This crowd is going insane!"

I rear back. Here's the moment I've been training for! My chance to finally draw back and unleash my *Rocky* punch.

"This is for killing the children!" I snarl and deliver an uppercut straight into The Big C's chin.

"There it is! That shot said lights out. Good night!"

The Big C's head jerks straight up. He stiffens. He topples backwards with a thud on the canvas. His legs shoot in the air. His shifting cells slowly transform him into a slag heap. His masked head snaps off his neck, thumps across the mat and the pulverized contents of what was once his skull, spills from his hood like brown sugar out of a split open five-pound sack.

My dying tumor has turned him inside out.

The commentator rabidly yells, "The Big C is down! It's pandemonium. The Big C is down! Forget about it. Not too many fighters can get up without a head. It's over! And this crowd. It's pure and utter pandemonium!"

I stand over the fallen champ and continue to count him out. "Eight. Who loves you? Nobody! Nine. You never fell in love, I have love! Ten. You're dead!"

"It's over, it's all over, The Chemo Kid has won the title and the Infusion Belt of champions!" declared the commentator. "This crowd has come to life!"

The sight of the vanquished tumor at my feet aroused a seething, exhilarating and glorious predatory fury within me. I flung off my gloves, growled, leaped and pounced on The Big C's disintegrating mound, growling and viciously raking my nails and clawing apart his dry rotted cellular compost.

There was one last thing to do. I sprung up, pull down my trunks, whip out my dick and pissed my name in his ashen remains.

"Yeah, that's who I am," I said. My cracked lips flash with the wide smile of eternity. I shoot my arms up in the air. "I'm still here!"

And our cats, Bogie, Groucho, and Brooksie appear, take my cue and use the ring containing The Big C's drying chunks as their personal litter box.

F-R-E-D! F-R-E-D! F-R-E-D!" chants the crowd.

I answer the crowd's cheers by exuberantly bellowing out one long ululating, triumphant, mean-ass cold-blooded lion-eating zebra roar.

All the music I've ever heard in my life resounds through the arena. My 57 Freds and everyone we've ever known, will know, and will never know, and loved and been loved by stormed through the ropes and joyously stomped and danced on The Big C's residue, kicking and scattering flakes of what's left of him into even smaller particles, like he was a blacken pile of burnt leaves.

"Today Cancer, tomorrow the world!" I proclaim as the rising and the fallen hold me up on their shoulders and walk within me to victory.

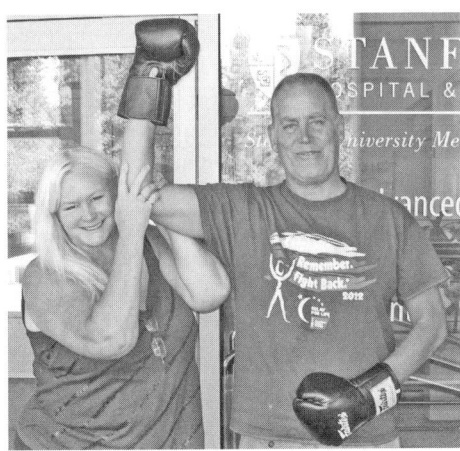

What's the point of knocking out cancer unless you win the girl?

NEGATIVE IS POSITIVE
GOT A *PROBLEM* WITH THAT?

THE DAY AFTER MY PET SCAN REVEALED NO SIGN OF CANCER, I got up at 5 A.M. of a new day. It's like being a kid on Christmas and under the tree was the best present I'd ever receive: my life. They say every day is a gift, right? I know why, I unwrap it every time I open my eyes. The difference is: for most people this is a motto, for me it's an *emotion*. Every time I blink I'm within a framed canvas watching another brush stroke being added to the painting. I've been told this euphoria tails off. Sure, I'll lose my ability to be mollified by shiny objects. Flip off a motorist who cuts me off, or get mad if I get treated rudely at work by a boss who knows I can't bark back because I need the job. But there is part of me the harsh world with never chill or bruise again. I'll find it amusing when someone attempts to make me feel less of myself, and realizes they can't leave a mark on me. They can't extinguish the spark in my eyes. The harder they try to smother me, the stronger and brighter I intensely burn and glow. My light will blind them. And by the time they regain their vision. I'm out of reach.

Later that day, I went to the closet and put on a Hawaiian shirt of an old friend who died from leukemia. When he died I was holding his ankles while his wife held his hands. His name was Mikel Herrington. He was a great original in radio. The film FM was based on his career as a program director in Los Angeles during the early '70s when radio was vibrant and fun. He created the KOME station in San Jose, CA ("Put a KOME on your dial."). Mikel was never very free with compliments. But once he said about my on-air talent, "Fred, I've only said this to a few people. But you're a natural." And because he said that to me, no critic or corporate suit who never cracked a mic and fired me could ever convince me otherwise. Mikel believed and admired and cultivated creative people and brought out the best in whoever was with him, he demanded it. He loved lighting the fuse to launch the talent and watch the glorious boom make the useless scatter and the cool applaud. Its call letters of an exploding light show attracted and guided and inspired the best. *I was faced with the responsibility of bringing out the best in me.* That's why I wanted to wear his shirt. It was like having his arm on my shoulder — he was proud of my ability to fight, and his spirit was pushing me along, like a christened boat. I imagined myself saying, "No, Mikel. You christened an iceberg looking for a ship to sink." I heard his rich, deep demonic laugh. I went outside cloaked by him to draw more sunlight.

As I walk, it's like I have gills and coasting beneath a surface. Everything is a flowing nectar warmly wrapping about me between two parallel worlds going in opposite directions. The ones who cling to the reality of death are no different to me than priests who desperately stroke the upraised blue-veined pole of celibacy as the whirling harem of life spins its cleavage around them. Their inevitable logic will come to pass, like sitting in the center of the merry-go-round where it doesn't move and reassured all rides inevitably stop so it validates their kinda lame all-is-vanity philosophy. Bring on the horses! Mount them with vanity plates! Bring on the spinning circles of going nowhere fast! Let's spin and spin. Death doesn't deserve extra credit. The people who use death as a contrast to appreciate life have never really seen it. That contrast never brings a moving picture into focus. After going through cancer and suffering and unable to dust off the pain of others, I seek sensations free of mortality. A second parallel world's unfurling and flapping moments of life that are an answer in themselves. It's like there's a film projector inside of me and I'm in my own movie where every camera shot and every second is a revelation and I star in the heating heart and moisture of me. I'm rolling till the film runs out. Life is a dream, and I guess it is if you're asleep the entire time you're here, but to me it's like everything we're seeing in front of us is broadcast from an antenna and we're receiving the signal. And this is as real as it gets. But that signal can vanish and then there's blackness and all that's left of us is a quivering white dot that defiantly remains on the screen and ideally we're going somewhere else.

It *had* to be this way. So much for self-fulfillment. I was broke, working part-time, looking for a dream. Now how the hell am I going to pay my hospital bills?

THE STANFORD HOSPITAL PICKS UP MY CANCER AND CHEMO TABS. I receive a financial reprieve from Stanford Hospital Patient Financial Services:

September 11, 2012,

Patient Name: Frederick Reiss
Medical Record Number: 25477894

Dear Mr. Reiss,
Thank you for completing and submitting a financial assistance application. Based on a review of the information you provided it has been determined that the patient listed above qualifies for financial assistance...has been approved to cover the patient liability due after insurance(s) pays their portion towards any Stanford Hospital Bills...

My running tab from my treatment escalated to over $70,000. And with future PET scans every three months and follow-up exams, testosterone fill-ups, six-dollar hospital garage parking fees, add another $30,006-plus. So, we're talking easily $100,006 and climbing. My health insurance covered the bulk of it, but I was still left with a significant future-numbed debt in the thousands, and now it was gone. I was lucky, but less fortunate without insurance spend the rest of their lives in a debtors prison without walls. Or are left to die.

I called the hospital and said, "I want to thank you. I lost my job and have been doing part-time work at wineries. I've kept up my medical insurance. My wife's really supported me otherwise I couldn't have made it this far. Having cancer blew me out of the water. I appreciate what you've done. And I don't want something for nothing. If there are people who have testicular cancer or are getting chemo and need someone to talk to, I'll be glad to volunteer and help."

I learned to be richer by wanting less and giving. But, it's a lot easier to be generous with your time when your mailbox isn't filled with bills you can't pay!

I WORE MY PURPLE HEART, HELD A BOX OF DOUGHNUTS AND STOOD WITHOUT TESTICLES IN MY END ZONE: the waiting lounge in the Stanford Cancer Center's Infusion Treatment Area. Last December, I stood here and received my chemo kick-off and did an open-field run through nine months worth of yardage to reach this destination. I wasn't here to showboat by spiking the ball and dancing in the end zone. To act like that is a sacrilege, really. There is a struggling holy somberness inside and outside this room that cries out for respect. If you failed to acknowledge the sanctity of their determination to live, you're defiling them. Near me was an old man in a wheelchair. He was distinguished looking, grief-stricken, had fixed flat-black eyes that looked like large dots of balsamic vinegar floating in olive oil. I knew what he was seeing: he was tumbling backwards without a chute into a widening, gulping pit. Through the windows that looked out into the gleaming tiled hallway illuminated by the sun from the vaulted ceiling's skylight was a Chemosabi lying on a flat cushioned bench, valiantly huddled under a blanket like a war casualty, and their weary and distraught caregiver sitting beside them doing a crossword puzzle. I knew their world. I had learned tears of pain and grief are salty and tears of joy are warm.

The waiting lounge was no longer a vacuum-sealed module. The air pressure inside the room was equalized to the air pressure outside. I traveled through one weightless galaxy and crossed over into a world of gravity and daylight savings. With each step, the room became more remote, as if I was walking away from it while I was still there. My illness was gone. *I've lost my sense of belonging.* I'm no longer compressed into the thick syrup of isolation. Its atmosphere evaporated. My chemo-soaked flesh was dried out. I'm outside the gravitational pull of their world. Nothing adhered to my resilience. My feet are back on Earth and the Chemosabis around me are adrift in this space station.

I'm a decommissioned Chemosabi with a mothballed fleet. I look like a visitor not a patient. I wasn't wearing any kind of hat. My hair had grown back. I was tan and filling out. I wore my Relay For Life purple T-shirt. Relay For Life holds volunteer/survivor runs to raise money for cancer. At the event Laurie released a dove representing my spirit. I was given a survivor T-shirt. I never expected the shirt to affect me so much. There's no denying it gave me an upwelling of pride and strength. It's my purple heart. Every time I come to the hospital it's my Veteran's Day. I was proud of the battle I fought. I wanted others at the Cancer Center to see my purple heart and know *there was a way out of here*.

The receptionist politely asks, "Can I help you?"

I want the Chemosabis in the waiting room to hear me and I loudly reply, "I got out of chemotherapy here three months ago, and they did a PET scan last week that said my cancer is gone. I made an appointment to get my Huber needle here for a blood draw, and then I go upstairs and get my port removed."

"That's wonderful," she says. I give her my name and birth date. She goes into the computer and states, "We don't have you in the system."

"I should be. My appointment at Interventional Radiology is in an hour."

"We'll try to work you in," she said, as if I was in a hair salon.

I notice some Chemosabis spot the words on the back of my T-shirt. Its writing states I'm a cancer survivor it. They knew I once sat in this room too — *I was once one of them.* I went down the hallway to the staff station. There were a couple nurses in the hallway, and others were in the break room behind the desk having lunch. I recognized a few but I didn't remember their names.

"Can I help you?" said the nurse behind the counter.

"I was here months ago and finished chemo," I replied.

The nurse studied me and narrowed her eyes, as if she was trying to remember the lurking memory of a thin and bald man beneath my healthy surface.

She nodded and said, "I remember you."

"I brought doughnuts," I said. "You guys were telling me to eat healthy but every time I brought doughnuts in, you guys powered them down. You guys eat crap."

A nurse opened the box, pointed at doughnut and said, "There's fiber in there. And coconut is a fruit."

"Look at your hair," said one of the nurses, rubbing my head. "It's coming back. It's curly. It's so soft! Like a baby's hair."

"Yeah, I know. I tell people to cop a feel all the time. When people ask me who does my hair, I say, 'The Stanford Cancer Center.' They laugh. "I say, 'They take seven months. It's very expensive. But it comes out fantastic!'" We laugh. "I'm getting all these compliments about having short hair from women. And women always know how a guy looks best. Anyone in their twenties tells me shorter hair makes me look younger. When I was growing up, longer hair was a statement of freedom because Vietnam hawks and rednecks had short hair. And why have short hair when you can grow it long? Seems like a waste. Kids associate short hair with being young because that's how they all look now. Their only frame of reference is themselves. All these women tell me to keep it short, so I guess I'll keep it shorter now. So I'll listen to that."

"You listen to women?"

"Yes, but I had to lose both testicles to hear them," I said, smiling.

"You've gained weight," said one.

"I would hope so. I lost over thirty pounds when I was here."

The nurses are getting busy. I excused myself and returned to the waiting room. Then I spot Molly, a young blonde oncology nurse, who I remembered because she was attentive and bright — and one of the many pretty nurses on the staff.

"Molly," I blurted. She peered for the thinner, flat-eyed me. "I was here a few months ago getting chemo." I see the relief of recognition forming in her face. "I have to wait out here to get my port connected. They don't know if they can fit me in."

Molly nods to the far door and says, "Come with me." We go to the blood drawing area. She sets up the needle and gauze and the tubes. There's a stocky, young Mexican guy with one leg getting chemo in the recliner next to mine.

"I brought doughnuts. You better hurry to get them. They go fast."

Molly nods then exits the room. I wait for a few minutes.

She returns, smiles and says, "I had one of the doughnuts."

"Good. That's what they're there for."

"You're giving back," observed Molly, unwrapping the packaging of the Huber needle. "There are many people who go through this, and so many come out of it wanting to give back."

"I suffered so much and saw so much suffering. I couldn't convince myself to feel sorry for myself. I tried, but it wasn't in me. I only felt the pain. Fought the pain. I just wanted to help others. The thing is I feel good, when you're sick, you're part of this whole place. But now I feel detached, I'm not in it anymore. I don't feel it. *But I know it.* I don't want to act too healthy in front of the people because it's subdued out there, and each person is an altar, and you have to respect that and genuflect in a way. Sometimes it's hard to believe this whole thing ever happened. Because once you're out of chemo, there's nothing similar to it in this world." My voice broke as I added, "Part of me will always be in that room. I can't leave them. I don't want to …"

She became pensive, nodded and said, "How long have you had this port?"

"I guess seven months. I didn't want to get it removed after chemo."

"And you finished chemo…"

"Three, maybe four months ago."

"Did you get it flushed every month?"

"No, I didn't want to come back here."

"You know they clot?"

"I figured I'd get lucky." I smiled. "I was due."

"Ready."

"I numbed it up so I'm all powerful."

She snapped a Huber needle into the port and said, "It worked."

"I thought so. I told you I was due for some luck! I didn't get the port removed after chemo. I wanted to make sure the PET scan showed I didn't have any cancer first. Removing it would be like being cocky and saying, 'I never get in car accidents' without knocking wood. I didn't want to defy fate. You gotta respect the thing that was inside you. I don't want to give it the impression I'm looking the other way."

"And you certainly don't want to go through having to get another port put in."

"That too," I said, watching her snap test tube after test tube onto the valve of the Huber needle and fill them with my blood.

"Does seeing your own blood bother you?"

"No," I replied, picking up one of the warm tubes. "It would bother me if I was *bleeding*. But when I've squeeze my own urine out of bags, you know, what can I say? Seeing blood in tubes is not a big deal. After chemo, my diet has changed. I still like wine and cocktails, but lost most of my desire for beer. My fridge always had a six-pack in it. And on a hot summer day I'd down beers. But that feel is gone. Now, I really like the taste of water! I'd never have water with meals, I do now. Can't handle fried foods anymore either, all I taste is oil."

"That's good."

"Sodas and junk food taste like chemicals. In the long run, it might change. But no desire, really."

"Maybe your body is telling you something."

"My body's been telling me way too much of something for a long time, let me tell you." I pause. "You know what really bugs me though? Clutter! I remember seeing my Nana in her room at an assisted living home. All her possessions had been narrowed down to photographs on the bureau. That stuck with me. Why hold onto stuff? At home I looked at my books and CDs. I removed any book I thought I'd eventually read but didn't from the shelves. And books I hadn't reread in years — well, time to pass them on. And music? Got rid of CDs I haven't even listened to for years. I went through my closet and thinned out my shirts as well as pants I'd never fit into again. I went through drawers and anything that has been in there and never used I threw away. I found about four new dental floss containers. I started giving things away to friends, selling stuff on eBay, or donating to Goodwill. So I buy new stuff. Keeping it fresh. And anything I kept for sentimental reasons, I put it in a place where I see it."

Molly labels my test tubes. I realize all I've done is talk about myself. I don't know anything about her except she, like all the nurses, helped me heal.

"So what made you become and oncology nurse?"

"Cancer affects a lot of different lives in different ways."

"Someone you knew?"

"My sister."

"Did she make it?"

"No."

"I'm sorry," I said. "Did you get to feel my hair?" She does. "I'm glad I saw you. There are nurses I remember but didn't see today."

"Not all of us are out in the hall. You can come back here and say hello to us."

"Okay, and I'll bring doughnuts," I said. "And life is treating you good?"

"Yes."

When I got up to leave, in the adjoining room I saw a Chemosabi in a recliner getting infused. It was the guy who was starting chemo the day I finished. He was completely bald and had a flat painted look on his face. He was initiated. Unfortunately, he *knew* what I knew. Welcome to the club. You're paying dues and never wanted to belong to it in the first place. But you're a member now.

ME UNPLUGGED: PULLING OUT OF PORT. I was in a hospital gown on a gurney, one of many patients separated from each other a station partitioned by curtains in the Stanford Cancer Center's Interventional Radiology clinic. I had been here before to receive my port. I had chemo side effects. The neuropathy felt like there was a wooden splint in my soles, and aching barnacles on the balls of my feet. My wrists throbbed with a prickling bracelet of clinging numbness. Today was cosmetic surgery, I wasn't being armed to handle chemo and needles, I was having my port removed, which was like pulling out a plug and disconnecting myself from the world of cancer, but it was more than that, it was like I was going to be recharged so I could run stronger my own power. The medical port under my skin above my collarbone was an essential part of my battle gear against The Big C. The port was the last thing that separated me from other civilians. It was like turning in your rifle before you're discharged from the service. My port was my best piece of combat equipment.

I was pleased again to meet the soft spoken Ryan Daugherty, the acute nurse practitioner who installed my port in January, and was removing it on this October day. His considerate behavior extended to our exit interview. He knew anyone who had a port hated needles, he spared me from an IV and used my port for the last time to keep me hydrated and administer sedatives.

"This port in the storm saved me," I said.

"So many people say it's their Teddy Bear," replied Ryan, who always made eye contact and tried to say everything in a gentle and soothing manner. "A lot of people who do it, regret they did it too late. They wish they did it earlier."

"You're right. My oncologist didn't give me any information about a port," I said. "I found out about it by talking to other chemo patients. They showed me how their veins were shot. When I was getting chemo, the ones I felt sorry for, were the people who only spoke Spanish. They're afraid. They don't know it's a simple operation that doesn't take that much time, and they don't put you under. Most people think surgery and see something complex. It doesn't have to be that way. What they should do is have a cardboard display with a port in English and Spanish in the waiting room of oncology that explains what it does. Because you're in shock when you find out you have cancer. So much of going through cancer is feeling like you're degraded — well, degraded is the wrong word. Your spirit is demoted into your body. The entire process dehumanizes you and takes you away from your life, and you need that spirit to fight. The less you get poked with needles, the more of you is left. The only people I didn't think highly of, are the oncologists because of their atrocious beside manners." I paused. "I'm sorry, I'm taking up your time."

"It's okay, this is your time, that's why I'm here," he said.

"See you're not like them."

"That's because I'm a nurse," he replied. "I sit at bedsides."

"Well, you are the guys who are *there*."

"A lot of people say what you say. These doctors go from school to school and become doctors without ever experiencing life. I've worked in hotels. I've had other jobs, dealt with people in different circumstances. These guys have never done another job. They've never been fired. That's why they don't have those skills." He paused for emphasis and said, "Still…" Then added in a wiser and deeper voice, "*What did yo' momma tell you?*'"

"You got that right," I said, smiling and nodding. "If they were raised to be a doctor, they should have also been raised to be a better person too."

Ryan's observation's also explained to me how the doctors could be so arrogant and inconsiderate and insensitive — they were nine-year old psyches encased in a big brain that never thought its spinal cord was connected to the nervous system of others. Sometimes if I dared question their intelligence and professional opinions and diagnostic abilities, I felt they were always on the verge of exploding into an over-educated tantrum.

"It's a simple procedure," said Ryan. "It'll take less than forty-five minutes."

"I figured it's like the difference between installing a CD player in your car, or stealing one," I said. "It always takes less time to rip it out."

Ryan excused himself and left. Here I was, back again at intermission. This is where the cancer-chemo ride began. And I reflected on my ride. I had woken up with catheters and urine bags. Saw my hair fall out in my hands. Couldn't eat because my mouth was rippling with sores. Lost weight. Was so weak I'd be out of breath after climbing five steps. Blacked out and fell on the bathroom floor. On a hot day, shivering in my defensive fetal chemo curl, bundled under layers and layers of blankets. It was hard to believe I persevered through all the needles and scans and exams and infusions, but I obviously went *through* something. When I was first here, this gurney was like a roller coaster car. I was restrained by the lapbar of circumstance. The chain-lift locked into it and I was dragged on a conveyor belt towards my cancer treatment and pulled upwards to a precipice and dropped. I was powered by momentum and gravity and not sure if I was falling to my death or winding on a track and building up speed to swoop back into life again. Here I was, almost a year later, the gurney had come to a stop, the lapbar was lifted off me, and I was hopefully at the end of the ride.

Through a narrow opening in the curtains that enclosed my area, I spotted a stricken woman in her thirties lying in a gurney. She was surrounded by distraught family members. Her face drained. Her brown eyes looked black and unreflective. I knew what it was like to nervously peer around those pupils. She was beginning her trip. I was on a different ride now — *forever, I hope.*

THEN AN HOUR LATER, I WAS OUT OF SURGERY IN POST-OP. All the nurses and attendants near me are upbeat. *A cured patient was leaving.* I was on chemo's catch-and-release program. My body was no longer cancer bait. The head-on force that didn't believe I could swerve made a powerful miss. I ran my hand below my collarbone. No bulge. Just a bandage. I didn't have a foreign object in me. I was like everyone else.

"Can I get you some juice or crackers?" asked a nurse.

"Oh. Just water, please," I said. "When I had my port first put in I thought apple juice was great. Now I can't stand it. And I really hate graham crackers. They gave them to us all the time in chemo. Hate them."

A stocky black attendant stood near me, listening and smiling. He was in his thirties. He thought my comments were funny. He seemed like a cool guy too.

The nurse said, "Do you want ice?"

"Yes please," I said. "What's your name?"

"Donna."

"Thank you."

The black attendant said, "I'll get your water." He took a few steps, turned and added, "Now, you're sure you don't want any apple juice, or graham crackers?"

I smiled and said, "You're busting me."

"I can get you graham crackers, really no trouble at all, we've got plenty of them they're by the apple juice," he said walking away, shaking his head and chuckling.

I smile and ask, "What's your name?"

"Joe."

"You're a funny guy Joe, I hope you die soon."

He laughs real loud.

Joe returns with the water. He watches me take a sip, then smiles and says, "Now, you're positive you don't want any *graham crackers* to go with that?"

We laugh.

"You know, I can get you some if you want one? We have lots of them. Really, it's no trouble," he chuckles. "I can get you extra graham crackers to eat on the way home. If you want to give me your address, I'll pack some up and mail them to you. You might want some later…"

I smirk. Amused to be back in a world that's still breaking my balls — *even though I don't have any!*

I CAN'T ALLOW CANCER TO DEFINE ME — if it does, I've given permission for the tumor to developed a second life. That's *not* why I fought The Big C. Cancer doesn't define a life. It *takes* life. I'm a veteran from the battle in the war against cancer. The experience can shape me, but I'm not a casualty, I'm a combatant, a victor. I can't allow cancer to become my life's frame of reference. I have to draw on the spirit within me and the loving support from people that enabled me to survive so I can relay that soulful glowing curing power to ignite others to win their battle. Oh, how I hope to keep this quiet fire alive for someone else.

"Cancer changed your life, but some people don't change," an oncology nurse once said to me. "You said the first time you had testicular cancer and it changed you. I find it's how people are raised. They respond to cancer proportionally the same way they act when they cut their finger or don't get their way."

I laughed. I found that funny.

The 1993 film *Fearless* depicts the dilemma of a cancer survivor, but the movie *isn't* about cancer. Jeff Bridges portrays Max Klein, a businessman who survives an airline disaster. When the plane is descending, Max peacefully accepts his death. The psychological trauma of survival alters his state of consciousness. In a key scene, a lawyer is trying to get Max to exaggerate his testimony to increase a widow's pain-and-suffering compensation from the airline. The widow is a wife of Max's friend, who died instantly in the crash. Max reluctantly agrees, then has a panic attack and bolts from the office to the roof of the building where he climbs onto the ledge, his arms extended, gazing upwards. Why? Max wants to recapture the fearless high he experienced during the crash. He doesn't want lying to contaminate that high — he might lose it! He needs the fearless adrenalin rush to avoid the sense of emptiness that is the form of death in life. Max says to others he's a ghost who "passed through death" by "touching the beauty" of existence and he doesn't "want to come back." Max desires to remain pure and states he "doesn't make sense and doesn't want to." No cancer survivor can maintain that same sensation and live day by day. It's suicidal. But you can't live every hour like it's your last. You can't remain in the afterglow of euphoric insights. You have to inhale the compromising fumes of the world. You have to come down from the summit into rush hour traffic and absorb and tolerate the lesser concerns and worries that preoccupy and absorb others. Restrain the joy as you struggle to do a caesarian on your squealing and squinting soul so you can pull out the best of your rebirth into the light of each day and accept it for what it is: a blessing that simultaneously haunts and drives you. Keep epiphanies to yourself. If you don't, you'll piss off others — or worse, bore them to death.

I wasn't immune from post-traumatic stress. I deluded myself into believing I was different because I could articulate my experience. I discovered this when leaving the house to work at a winery tasting room.

"If you want to work out other living arrangements we can," said Laurie.

"What are you talking about?" I snapped. Her comment came out of nowhere. It pissed me off.

"You don't seem to be happy here," she said. "You snap at me all the time."

"No I don't," I snapped. "I have to go to the winery, and I don't want to be late, and you're bringing this crap up now. Great way to start my day."

"I'm trying to —"

"Big help, try something else. Thanks."

I stomped out of the house and drove to work. My brow was furrowed. I was scowling. My eyes were hard. I got in the car and sped off. Anger welled up inside me. I couldn't control it. *I liked it because I believed I was right.* Then I remembered when I first experienced this rage. Fred-27 had testicular cancer and finished radiation for the day. I sat in a kitchen and I said to my sister Cindy, "It's very difficult going through this." She mimicked me and said, "It's very difficult going through this." I became enraged. I threw her down on the kitchen floor and kicked her several times in the ass. Then I stormed out, drove away. I completely lost it. That had never happened to me before. I was mortified. I pulled over to a phone booth and called Cindy back. I was crying and said, "I'm sorry I did that. I lost control. I must have everything a certain way. And if it goes another way, I lose it. I'm sorry. You have to understand. I'm sorry." She said, "It's okay. I shouldn't have said what I said. Why don't you come back for some coffee?" I returned and we ate breakfast. Cindy was nicer then. I wasn't.

I drove through the Santa Cruz Mountains to Beauregard Vineyards in Bonny Doon. I snarlingly mulled over what Laurie said to me. I didn't feel bad about a single thing I said to her. *That was the problem.* I was insensitive. I thought about how I went off at the beach on the Spandex macho guy with the dogs. I was still armored in a protective shell, distrustful of any outside influences, hunkered down to fight cancer in my machine gun nest. I didn't stop firing at any emotion that broke my concentration to defend my new life. Now, my chemo curl was unwinding in the opposite direction, whipping and lashing out at life not cancer. This gnashing rage hurt Laurie. I couldn't even tell you what I said, because I was completely unaware I was doing it because I didn't care. I felt completely justified by my actions — *and that should have been the warning sign.* This realization collapsed the walls separating the survivor and the cancer fighter. A spiky foiled cloud crunched inside me, singed my eyes, and I began crying.

I saw a defiant biker drive in the opposite direction on the road, dressed in camouflaged clothing. A bearded guy with a braided ponytail. No sleeves on his shirt. His muscular arms were heavily tattooed with angry skulls and snakes and flames. Obviously, a Vietnam veteran in his mid-sixties. A pole rose from the sissy bar on the back of the cycle's seat, flying a ridiculously huge black MIA flag. He was a parade of justified self-righteousness, trying to provoke people, and clearly ready to punch anyone who disrespected his service. I vividly remembered the generational strife and divisiveness during that period. Oddly, the time-is-now generation that largely prided itself on its refusal to acknowledge history wanted to be remembered as history. Hey, I'm not belittling them or their sacrifice. But a lot of those guys were drafted and didn't want to be in the war. I could easily understand conflicted pride. I felt like a veteran from a battle too. We'd been in different firefights where we saw our death and the death of others, and the wounds, too many wounds. But Veteran's Day is still only one day. Some people make it 24 – 7 – 365. The biker remained uniformed and locked and loaded with every clenched argument to validate himself. Maybe he was still angry someone sent him who didn't serve and he didn't want anyone with a deferment to forget or forgive their offense for all the deaths. This guy made me realize I was also a walking armored vehicle always on the ready to respond to any potential trespassing slight by spinning my head like a turret to flash a repelling glare and fire a sharp remark. I was MIA because I thought I built a fortress, but really constructed a penitentiary where I imprisoned in solitary confinement. I didn't want to end up like that vet on the motorcycle, no longer able to tell the difference between incoming and an extended hand of help. You have to be bigger than the battle you fought to overcome your war.

Cancer rearranged the furniture of my life, and I can't fit all of it back into my room again. So I have to leave it behind. Maybe it's meant for someone else now.

I called Laurie on my cell phone, hysterically sobbing and said, "I'm sorry I didn't know I was acting like that. I love you and I'm sorry. Tell me whenever I do it and I won't do it anymore." My lips trembled. "I'm sorry."

"It's okay," she said, upset I was so panicked.

I squeezed through the perforated stitches of the wound binding my two worlds. It was safe to have an open border. But inside me, a sentinel was keeping watch over The Big C's incinerated remains, standing guard over the an extinguished pyre, making absolutely certain there is no sign of any glowing metastasizing embers to combust into a blaze. The sentry was primed to kill any sign of cancer kindling to life. That's where my new imaginary veteran belonged, stationed and armed but only facing the direction of the entombed tumor not life. He'd always remain at his post, but I can't allow my keeper to stick his jutting bayonet between me and the outside world again.

After work, I returned home, I saw Laurie, smiled and cheerfully said, "Hi! How are you?"

I meant it.

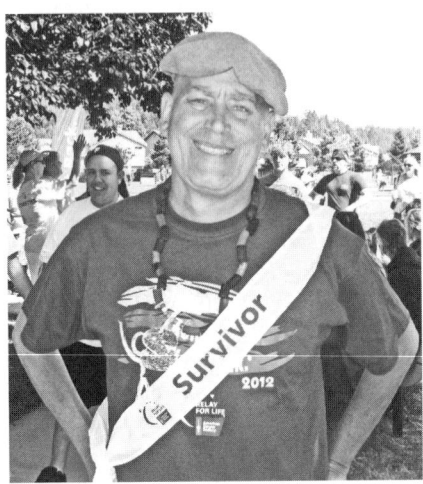

THERE'S A KEY DISTINCTION THAT RANKS CANCER SURVIVORS APART BUT NOT ABOVE OTHERS. Most people cruise life's highway. They're rapidly continuing on their journey to save time. Cancer survivors drive in a different lane with an inevitable toll plaza looming ahead of us. I slow at the approaching sight of blinking red lights and pull into a cylindrical front-loading white tollbooth. A gate lowers to prevent me from speeding through it. I stop, toss my hope and soul into the toll's copay receptacle basket. I'm lanced with PET/CT scan radiation. Is cancer dead or making a comeback? I stare at the lowered gate and await the test results to declare I'm still free from cancer's choke hold. I'm jittery. The gate must rise. Then and only then will I be allowed to continue my journey. But what if it doesn't? Will I be remanded into chemo custody?

Tears roll as I stammer between gasps, "Please, I don't want to get sick again. I don't want to get sick again."

The gate rises — this time.

When cancer survivors drive through the toll, the unimpaired carefree are irritated. We aren't going fast enough to merge back into the human race of life's highway. We're slowing them down. They honk, pass us and grumble, "While we're young!" After all, they have things to do, places to see. We don't mind. We pull over and let them speed by. Why get into with them? There are too many flowers blooming for us to dance among the weeds. We protectively brake to allow reflection, wisdom, judgment and innocence to safely make it across the road. We're riding with the top down to feel the warm highs, taking in the scenery of quiet moments of exhilaration with a different kind of slowed-down acceleration. The passing of time doesn't steal our enjoyment. And sometimes we happily cry too much on beautiful days — and there's a beautiful every second.

We're an equation that resolves itself. For our tentative lives are but gliding inflections in this wonderful jet stream. We're effortlessly doing chin-ups on the horizon. Isn't it wonderful living up to just being you? Surviving cancer *inserts* you into a different totality of perpetuality. You're ultra sensitive and dialed into every moment. Bland colors acquire sheen. Shallow values have a deep section. You pick up every distinct aroma, spice, daydream, drum beat, and the crisp nippiness in every blade of grass. Every day is a life resurfaced. You're a walking palette that tastes beyond sweet and sour. You see deeper into darkened rooms. There's more warmth from the sun on overcast days. You're fascinated while others are bored. In the middle of the night, you don't mind being unable to get back to sleep. Why? Because you're *here*.

When you're fighting cancer gently swaying filaments of sensitivity extend from every pore and hair follicle of your body. *But as you heal*, these highly reactive filaments retract. Everything is reversed. Instead of fighting to remain alive, you have to live in the world. Every color, breeze, and breath, drifts its filaments *towards you*, but you have to give of yourself to feel them. The dreamless people don't have those filaments. They have tentacles to catch prey, so every new sensation is paralyzed by their bitterness. The blunted who learned nothing from surviving cancer, leave the hospital with sharp quills of resentment pointing inward from every pore. They are armed against themselves. Too dumb to see their own karma. Their self-inflicted lives are their punishment. But the fortunate ones stung into action by seeing and feeling the suffering of others are anointed with the haunted blessing of being baptized and cursed by The Big C and emerge into a vibrant flavor-enriched world with wisps of chilling emptiness that compels us to run faster toward our overheating hearts to fill the void. Tell us life is meaningless and our souls will form a tight hard fist that blossoms into an extended open warm and soft palm to help others across the unsteady dance floor of whatever comes next.

All we can hope for is a Fast Pass to clear the many checkpoints ahead.

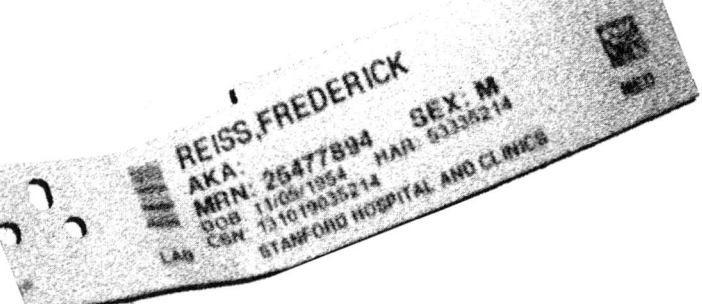

AND IN THE END...

I'M MARCHING ON MY CANCER-FREE PARADE ROUTE THROUGH OUR SANTA CRUZ MOUNTAIN NEIGHBORHOOD. It's twilight. Indian summer. The orange sun slants through the redwoods. I'm wearing headphones and timing my scenic route to the perfect second side of The Beatles remastered *Abbey Road*. Throughout chemo I listened to The Beatles music in chronological order (I skipped *Yesterday* because the song is sulky and depressing — I believe life can be changed for the better every day. No one should be fixed by the compass of the past. I also eliminated *Revolution Number 9* from *The White Album* — it sucks, along with *She's Leaving Home* on *Sergeant Pepper* due to the stupid harp.). The Beatles. Impossible to ignore their significance — even if you feel they didn't shape you, they shaped everyone else, so you're influenced by them whether you liked them or not — even today! Fred-9 first heard the Fab Four on a transistor radio in our next-door neighbor's front yard when I lived at 57 Sherman Place, Clifton, New Jersey. A group of teenage girls were smiling and laughing and dancing to *She Loves You*. The Beatles are a must to time travel into various periods of my life. The music was a melodious apron of a spreading gulf stream to a warming future. And tonight, I was slipping back into the familiar current of their Liverpool groove to sail home.

This remastered *Abbey Road* bursts and sprouts hundreds of new notes and arrangements and interwoven harmonies and lyrics I've never heard before! Every song is a liquid poem I'm swimming through this settling evening. People driving by me spot a grown man carrying a flashlight, wearing headphones and connected to an iPod, who occasionally does a little dance. They don't realize I'm marching with a baton not a flashlight. And I'm not alone. I'm alongside my 57 Freds in our big V-J Cancer Day ticker-tape parade. Our arms upraised and hands shaking in a hallelujah chorus of freedom and leaving a fertile vapor trail of Mom and Dad and family and all my friends and neighbors and caregivers and all the ghosts of relatives and people who built me from the inside out while I wasn't looking and all the girls I knew and never knew and the best and worst of my past, combining their total force to expand a propulsive energy rush to a regretless future. Our processions is on a roll! Everything else, the self-inflicted wounds of slights, grief, disappointments, judgments, professional failings are dissolving like stitches that no longer leave a scar.

But there is someone else.

He's still thin and gaunt and in a hospital gown. He's the teenager with the brain tumor who I met over thirty years ago at the Norwalk Hospital. He dreamed of becoming a photographer. He didn't make it. But he followed me with his haunting chant: *Live your dreams, the dreams I can't have*. He's been foreman of my jury ever since. I imagine him nodding, pulling out a camera and snapping a picture. He flashes a thumbs up. He disappears. He's letting me go on my own recognizance. He's found me innocent.

My soul burst. A tingling wave peaked and sprayed through my head, receded backwashed upwelled within my skull and effervescently crashed and soaked me. I surfaced from it, dripping broke, with nerve damage, ringing ears, no prospects, no testicles. If my new life is a fresh puzzle, I'll pick up its pieces from chemo's ocean floor and assemble them into a book to help people. That's where I'll begin to solve it. Let's see where this recast Fred-57 leads me. I stop and address all my Freds, "Have I become the Fred you wanted us to be?" And my remark is met by silence because the answer is obvious. I smile and add, "Dumb question, it's not like we have a choice. After all, he got us this far!" We laugh. I cried and clamped my lips tightly together. All the Ages of Fred and friends and lovers and memories ricochet off flashbacks as they soak into my body, fade, and synchronize. And I continue our one-man band on the parade route we've followed out entire lives, ignoring the street signs and concrete directions and reconfigured financial judgments of the dreamless others and blindly go off road guided by highly questionable one-liners and footwork.

I pass my next-door neighbor's house. He's away. Tomorrow is garbage day. We had our differences because he encroached on our property line. I pulled out the garbage, then looked at his trash can. I had every reason not to be nice. A force intravenously pulsed through me, dripping from an invisible tube connected to a bag of glowing energy. Reverse chemo. Its dose bored through me. I knew its welcome appearance would come again and I'd draw on its unpredictable life-altering presence throughout my life. It said why be right? Be bigger than me.

So, I pulled my neighbor's garbage out in the street, stood at the cans and looked up with tear-tinged eyes for approval from The Great Unknown, smiled and said, "Learning! See me? I'm learning.. I'm *better!* I learned something didn't I? Didn't I?" I laughed, regained my composure, and added, "Why am I talking to you? Throughout all I've gone through so far, you've never been very good about holding up your end of the conversation." And I laughed louder.

When Fred-27 had cancer he decided to change my life. Guess what? He did! And it worked! Outside of not going to Australia, I achieved every personal goal I desired without really earning anything at the expense of others. Maybe, that's why the shadow I cast doesn't have a mortgage. Never having gone to Australia isn't a big deal. After all I've gone through, every time I blink I travel around the world. What others have done for me is a journey. The first time cancer changed my life. Now I'm more tightly connected to how the immeasurable wonder of giving multiplies and divides and rushes back faster than you can receive and I splash its overflow and spray to the wind and enjoy the refreshing breeze as it blows back healing smiles in my face. I've been blessed twice. I don't want to get too weird about it. I'm no saint, and I never want to be one. But I go out of my way more for others, pass on things I use to people, listen longer than talk, hold eye contact, ask a stranger how their day is going, give gifts to others for no reason, tip more, leave a extra food on my plate for the pets, and try to linger as long as I can within sustained moments. I'm happily caught up in the gravitational pull in the world of giving back. There's no way I can be overdrawn in that account. It's a debt I can live with forever.

I descend three flights of stairs from the road, holding the railing to keep my balance on my numbed and prickling feet, which feel more like rockers attached to my ankles. I teeter and tilt, smiling.

Ringo's drumming launches *Abbey Road* into *The End* and The Beatles sing:

Oh yeah, all right.
Are you going to be in my dreams tonight?

Before I go inside, I walk past my new surfboard on the deck to the railing and check on the cactus in the Popeye Spinach can. The little guy has grown taller, greener, and has a wider fan of purplish-tinged leaves. My buddy is thriving. I feel the identical shape of his expanding growth tingling in the center of my pelvic region. I knew why I was upset when he was uprooted and dying, and why I desperately wanted to save him. My green budding buddy. The little guy represented *my growing hope*. And here we are, together again.

"Hey pal, how you doing?" I said fondly, picking up the can.

I smiled, put the plant down and looked at our house. I thought of my younger Mom and Dad in our new home in Freehold, New Jersey. I bet some nights they had their arms around each other and softly stepped down the hallways and peered through the open doors of my room, along with the rooms of my brother, and two sisters. I could easily see Dad wondering how he got here and laughing and Mom shaking her head in affectionate amusement at this odd man she loved. Their spirits had given me this ability to sustain this life and find my way back through the help of everyone else I met along the way. I was at the end as well as the beginning of a long receiving line.

I spoke to them from a pointed timid ecstasy, "Mom, Dad, I wish I knew as a kid what I know now so I could go back and make you *happier*." My face clenched and puckered as warm tears pooled in the corner pockets of my eyes. I dryly croaked, and gasped the words out, "But... you still came to... *save me*...thank you."

I perfectly timed entering our home as The Beatles sang their final:

> And in the end.
> The love you take is equal to the love you make.

I removed the headphones and quickly wiped away my tears. I didn't want Laurie to worry about me. She's busy and doesn't notice.

She putting cat food in bowls. "Did you see what's over there? It came today."

On the table is a Sorrento's Sub sent to me from Freehold, New Jersey. *The Number 5 Super*: provolone cheese, salami, boiled ham, capicola, prosciutino. Frank Doyle, a close friend from our old neighborhood, overnighted the sub to me. We grew up mainlining those Number-5 Supers. They reinforced a Jersey rebar within our spines. No sub since has ever tasted better to me. There's a deliciously spectacular culinary power of East Coast bread and beefsteak tomatoes and shredded lettuce slathered in a oils with mounds of wildly unwholesome thick and fat entrenched cold cuts. I hoist the sub up. Its saturated heft sags at the ends. The sub's dampened and slightly soggy and pinched sides are overlapped with unevenly slapped together slices of layered meats tinged with the peppered edged with Capicola and wedged with provolone cheese.

But before I took a bite of the sandwich, I needed to create the appropriate Jersey atmosphere. I went to the closet, put on my red Sorrento's Sub T-shirt, then grabbed a CD, cranked up our stereo and set the mood with Bruce Juice: Springsteen's *Tenth Avenue Freezeout*.

I sat at the table, deeply inhaled the Sorrento sub's oils, and tore off a bite of the sandwich. The sub was more than everything I wanted it to be — *it was the greatest bite I'd ever take in my life*. It was like receiving holy communion without ever having to confess because your sins are so damn original. I savored the past with the meal of the present. I ate comfort food from the home town that fed my hungry soul. My taste buds were returning the flavor of me.

I hear a mea-yap. Bogie is sitting at my feet, looking up and making direct eye contact, expectantly wobbling his head from side to side. All twenty-three pounds of him wants pets. And he wants them now. I laugh. We've both been rescued by strangers who became lovers. I pick up Bogie and wrap him around my neck. His black fur is so smooth. He's like a mink stole with soft paws.

"Who's the biggest little guy, Bogie? You're the biggest little guy," I say to him and laugh as Bogie chews, purrs and nurses on my ear lobe. "Who got better Bogie? We got *better* Bogie. We got better."

Slowly, the Earth begins to settle and revolve.

My flattened world is round again.

It's nice to know even cancer makes *some* things possible.

And that's as real as it gets.

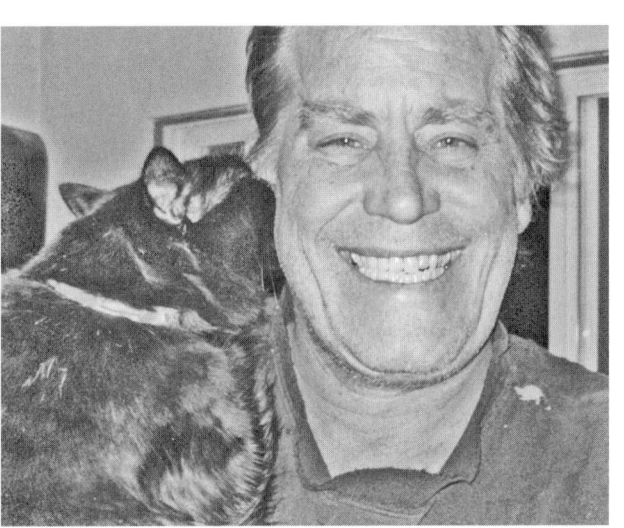

FRED'S CHEMO CLIFF NOTES

HERE ARE FRED'S CHEMO CLIFF NOTES. Before I finished this volume, I sent a letter with these suggestions to the head of the Stanford Hospital's Cancer Center, Mr. Amir Dan Rubin. My goal was to make it easier on the next person going through chemo, possibly help relieve their suffering, and improve their care. A few weeks later, I received a call from Terry Doyle, Stanford Hospital Disease Management Group Operations Manager. A dedicated and conscientious guy.

"Fred," Terry said. "I want to tell you, your suggestions are valid, and we're going to take steps to implement them. I'm an administrator. But you — you went through the fire and came out of it. They can't ignore you."

I added this section so people can easily glean tips to help others going through chemo and cancer as well as ways for patients, and oncologists to improve their care and attitude to fight The Big C.

Let's hope hospitals seeing this list move ahead and act on it, and don't get mired in committee meetings and legal. Be a hero to the suffering, just do it!

TIPS FOR ONCOLOGISTS OR DOCTORS

- Call patient's immediately with the results of their tests.

- Inform patients chemo also goes after the nervous system. Perhaps, add mineral or glutamine to their chemo hydration to reduce the effects of neuropathy.

- Ask a patient where they're from or their profession so they remember who they are, instead of what they've been reduced to.

O ncologist give patients the option of a medical port! Pictured here: two great healers (You can always tell a true healer by their eyes.): acute nurse practitioner Ryan Daugherty, holding a medical port, with a cute registered nurse, Courtnie Defigueiredo.

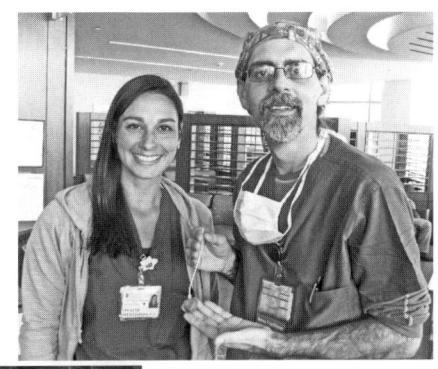

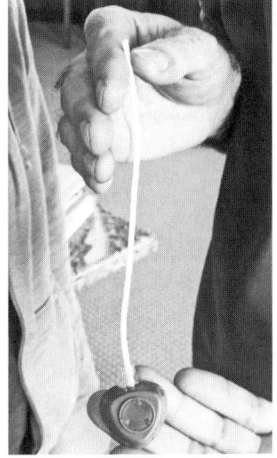

TIPS FOR ONCOLOGISTS OR DOCTORS

- If a patient requires chemotherapy and doesn't like needles — who does? — inform them about a medical port (*See above.*). Demonstrate the device. Explain it's *simple* surgery. (An objection oncologist have: you can get infections from a port. Well, you can *also* get infections from IVs and nurses can be off some days sticking a vein.). Provide a port brochure at patient's first appointment. **Muy Importante:** Some patients don't speak English, have a translator explain a port — I saw many of these people with bruised veins and who didn't know about ports.

- Don't expect the patient to ask correct questions. They're in shock, you're not. It's an exam not a test! Give them the answers before they ask the questions.

- Explain why you became an oncologist.

- Before a patient goes through chemo, conduct a hearing test. So after they finish chemo you can discover if they suffered hearing loss.

TIPS FOR ONCOLOGISTS OR DOCTORS (CONT.)

- After a patient is done with a procedure, write a release order as quickly as possible so the IV can immediately be taken out of their arm.

- Acknowledge high medical costs and tell the patient they will get bills and calls from collection agencies but the hospital offers financial assistance for them.

- **Don't do this with a patient's file: 1.)** address a patient while holding up their file. **2.)** look down at a file when you tell the patient the results of a test.
  Try this: Go over a file by placing it between you and the patient like you're both sharing homework — you know, working together?

- Instead of weighing people in kilograms and explaining tumor size in centimeters, use pounds and inches. I mean you bill us in dollars and cents. Describe tumor size as an object, like a baseball or an HMO executive's conscience?

- Remember just because you were "out of clinic" that day the patient was "in clinic." If you can't be there, make sure someone else can provide test results — or, tell the patient in advance who they can directly call for the information.

- Give your patient an option of preventative medicines *before* they suffer chemo's side effects, such as mouthwash rinses or numbing gels to alleviate sores.

- Don't want to take your work home? Why? Patients *take* your work home.

- Imagine the patient is in your family. Or, someone you care for the most.

- **Don't ask chemo patients, "How are you feeling?" Try this approach: 1.)** "Have you been able to eat?" **2.)** "Are you able to sleep?" **3.)** "What fluids besides water can you drink?" **4.)** "What activities have you been able to do, or miss?" **5.)** "When do you experience the most pain after you leave here?" **6.)** "Is there a term I used or something you don't understand?" **7.)** "What are you worried the most about in your treatment?"

- Personally call the patient at home if: **1.)** There's a change in medication. **2.)** They've completed a chemo cycle. **3.)** During chemo recovery week to ask how they're doing.

- It's hard seeing cancer patients, but you're a healer. A wondrous gift. Healing *requires* creating a caring relationship with the patient.

- When you see a patient wheeled on a gurney in the hallway, get out of the way!

TIPS FOR ONCOLOGISTS OR DOCTORS (CONT.)

- Visit patients in Infusion for support: **1.)** on first day of chemo. **2.)** on last day of chemo. **3.)** to remind yourself of their suffering so you can learn to improve your care.

- Talk and listen to the oncology nurses more often, and go out of your way to acknowledge and appreciate their views — plus, reach into your pocket and buy them some doughnuts or chocolate once in awhile. Remember, they have *better* people skills than you — you have many things to learn from them.

- Know your place. You chose to be a doctor. The patient didn't choose to have cancer. They *outrank* you.

HOW CHEMO PATIENTS CAN IMPROVE THEIR ATTITUDE AND CARE

- Remember you have cancer. Cancer doesn't have you.

- See The Infusion Treatment Area as a Fitness Center to get stronger.

- Chemo has a half-life. You have a *full* life.

- Don't play victim. You know when you fight cancer? When you agree to treatment. So when you lose hair, get nauseous, get fatigued, don't view the side effects as unfair, see them as a result of a *choice you made to get better.*

- Talk to other people who went through chemo before you take chemo. They can give you invaluable advice on foods, side effects or questions to ask.

- Before you go in for your appointment, make a list of questions with a friend or advocate, and have them ask those questions to the oncologist.

- Trust your instincts, if you don't like your oncologist's attitude or aren't pleased with your care, address those issues or request another oncologist.

- When doctors meet to discuss your case, such as at a Tumor Board hearing, *you have a right to attend it.*

- You always have the right to a second opinion.

- Before you brush your teeth, run the toothbrush under hot water, it softens the bristles so your gums won't hurt or bleed as much.

- People want to help you, it's part of their therapy too, so let them give.

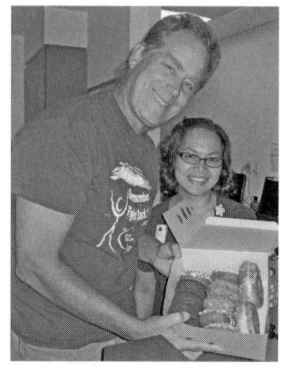

When you go for chemo bring doughnuts for the nurses. They care for you. Show you care for them. Give them the crap food they crave! After you finish your chemo, return and bring them goodies. Build up your good karma points to keep cancer away.

HOW CHEMO PATIENTS CAN IMPROVE THEIR ATTITUDE AND CARE (CONT.)

- While getting chemo, go through each year of your life, and imagine each year is a person on your side, along with all the people you knew then.

- Decorate your recliner with blankets, scarves, anything upbeat, bright.

- Visualize the tumor as a monster and fighting it.

- Don't feel bad about losing your hair and weight — appearance belongs to another world, clinging to those looks is denial. Accept your new look.

- If you can't read, listened to books on CD or watch DVDs.

- Bring doughnuts or treats for the nurses (**See above.**).

- Chemo's effects can be brutal. Ask your caregiver if you hurt their feelings by snapping at them. Remember, they are upset to see you suffer.

- Your life is best weapon against cancer, don't forget who you are.

- A nausea warning sign is burping. Take a pill quickly!

- If you have an iPod load it with the music that emotionally inspires you.

- **Besides mine, read these books:** Robert Schimmel, *Cancer on $5 (Chemo Not Included We The Victors* by Curtis Bill Pepper, and *A Taste of My Own Medicine* by Dr. Edward E. Rosenbaum. (If the books are out-of-print, get used copies online.)

- Never hesitate with medications, when in doubt, stay ahead of the pain.

Thank Your Caregivers!

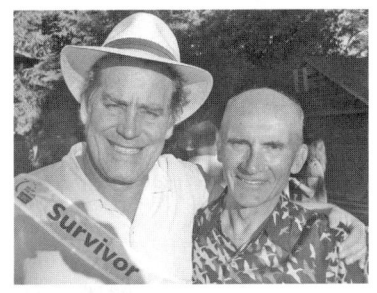

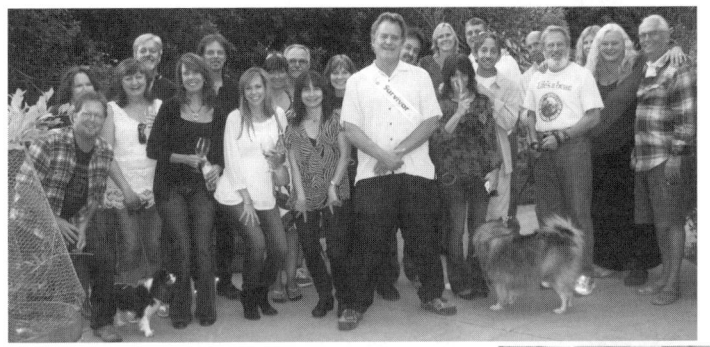

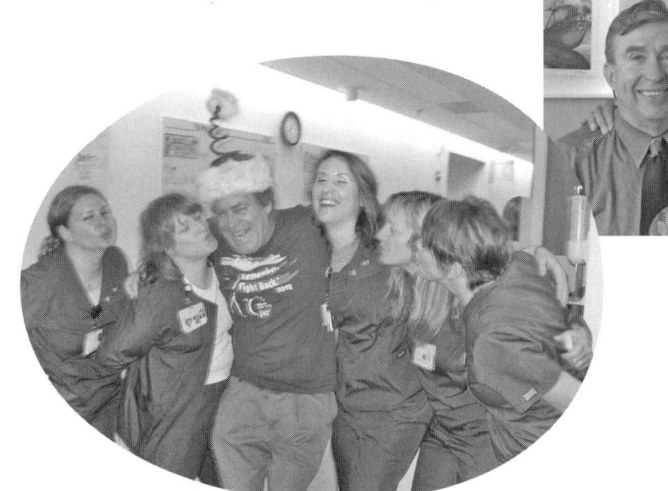

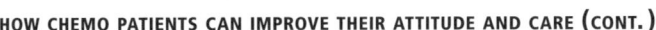

HOW CHEMO PATIENTS CAN IMPROVE THEIR ATTITUDE AND CARE (CONT.)

- You can be alone, beat cancer and survive, but you can't defeat cancer alone and *have* a life. So throw a party for your caregivers. **Top:** Dr. David Resnick-Sannes of Scotts Valley, CA, who saved my life. **Left:** A few of my many caregivers (the rest were drinking in the wine cellar of the Hallcrest Winery in Felton.). **Right:** Dr. Zen Majuk of Santa Cruz, he's everything his name represents. He guided me. **Bottom:** the stellar oncology nurses at the Stanford Cancer Center on Christmas 2012 (I brought them candy, peanut brittle, xmas music, and caramels for the patients.). They helped me take more from cancer than it could get from me.

HOW CHEMO PATIENTS CAN IMPROVE THEIR ATTITUDE AND CARE (CONT.)

- When you leave the hospital, don't think about it. When you're home think about everything else.

- Don't see chemo as a poison. See it as a serum. Let cancer see it as a poison!

- Get a DVD copy of *The Doctor* (An uplifting drama about cancer.).

- Even if you feel good, *always* take the anti-nausea medicines.

- No matter how smart or arrogant and intimidating a doctor can be, *they still work for you.* They're your employee, but try to be a good patient.

- Watch your favorite movies to remind yourself of your dreams.

- Try to find humor in your situation *(See opposite page.)*.

- You can't cure yourself, but you can insist on ways to *relieve* your pain.

- Don't say in self-pity: 'How could this happen to me?" or "Why Me?" or "This isn't fair." Your anger must be *directed at cancer not your situation.*

- Ask the nurses why they chose oncology. Most do this work because someone close to them had cancer. They're dedicated people.

- Find a stylish hat and wear it to your chemo — only wear a knit cap at home to stay warm, but don't wear a knit cap at the hospital, stand out!

- Dress in nice clean clothes, stay away from drawstring pants.

- Keep a journal, blog or *Facebook* page. You'll get feedback and support from others who have cancer, or know someone who had or has cancer or lost someone from it.

- When getting chemo surround yourself with Get-Well cards, pictures from your life or watch photos from your life as a slideshow on your laptop.

- If you can, make an effort to talk to other patients.

- Before you go to the hospital make sure insurance approved your procedure or the new drug you were scheduled to receive at your appointment.

- See everything you're going through as a path to a cure.

Stanford Cancer Center Intravenous Salon
Chemo Hair Club & Weight Loss Program
Perfect Color and Fit Cut.
Looking to lose 30 to 40 pounds?

Choose from our variety of Chemo-friendly styles!

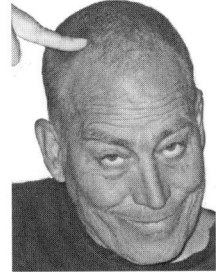 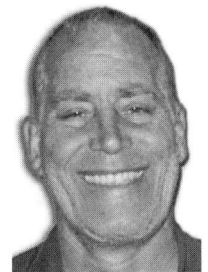 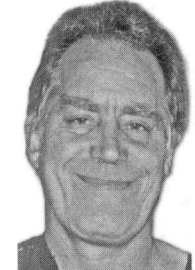

Skateboarding Stoner   Cheerful Roofer   Starfleet Commander

Become cancer free! Get kinky, luxurious, baby-soft hair with more body! We make foods you once loved *taste so bad* you're positively *guaranteed* to lose weight!

Your Cost only $70,000 – $100,000!**

At **SCCIS's** clinical salon infusion-based clients receive the latest technology in four-week treatments* custom-made to their specific needs by our in-house Oncology Tumor Stylist. Includes daily chemo-soaking intravenous drips with saline hydration and remission conditioners. Enjoy our all-you-can-eat buffet of saltines and graham crackers! Free water and juices. Begin your session with complimentary vital sign readings. Record your urine flows. Enter our blood drawing raffle. Infusion beauty pain-management side effects may include nausea, hearing loss, nerve damage, sores, infections and fatigue due to white and red blood cell reduction. But "prolonging the quality your hair's life" is worth it!

*Some programs last indefinitely and may require treatment at our radiation spa.

**Costs vary if your insurance provider denies coverage to cure you.

HOW CHEMO PATIENTS CAN IMPROVE THEIR ATTITUDE AND CARE (CONT.)

- Take photographs of yourself throughout your treatment (*See below.*). If you're trying to preserve a memory that means you will reach a day to look back on it.

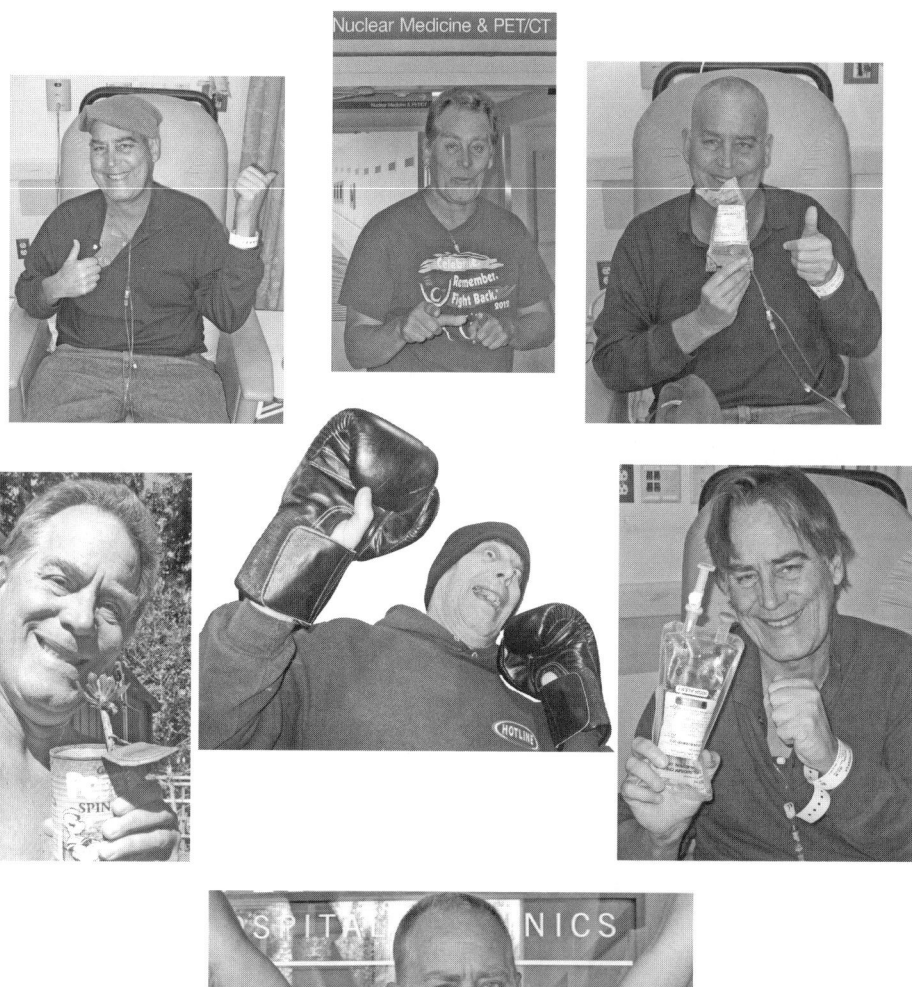

CHEMO FOOD TIPS

- Use plastic utensils to reduce the metallic taste of chemo's side effects.

- Don't try your favorite foods, or you'll never want to eat those dishes again.

- Fudge with hash, or marijuana-buttered cookies will help you sleep.

- If you find a food or drink you like, don't buy a lot of it, the next day you might be repulsed by it.

- If there's a sauce you like, such as barbecue sauce, slather your food with it.

- Imagine eating your favorite meals so you have a menu goal. That way, instead of being bummed by chemo, you're thinking towards a future of getting healthy.

- Ask oncology nurses what foods to eat during chemo, or ask other patients.

- If you find a food that tastes like it looks, stick with it — it's like being back in the world.

- Smoke marijuana before you eat — it'll animate some fragments of taste.

- **Try these foods:** Soft vanilla ice cream cones, Carnation Instant Breakfasts (Chocolate, Vanilla, Strawberry.), soggy Wheaties or other cereals, like Puffed Rice or Puffed Wheat, caramels, salted bagels pretzels (as well as ones with peanut butter inside), popsicles, Creamsicles, Fudgsicles, fruit bars, spicy foods, sushi with wasabi,* pork ribs covered with sauce, ice tea, peanut butter out of the jar, Gatorade protein & vegetable & fruit drinks (Fruits could hurt if you have sores.), oatmeal with brown sugar or cinnamon, tops of blueberry muffins, soups (tomato, sweet-and-sour, miso, tortilla).

*They warned me raw fish could lead to bacterial infections. And warn you about spicy. But I figured I'm soaked with chemo, who the hell cares? Eating gave me the will to live.

HOW HOSPITALS CAN IMPROVE INFUSION TREATMENT AREAS

- Instead of having professional nutritionists or counselors, hire a cancer survivors to do those jobs. Their advice would be more effective and taken more seriously.

- Have pictures in the hallway of people who survived cancer: or, a binder in the lobby with pictures of survivors and letters from them (Hey, bed and breakfast places do this, why not Infusion Clinics?).

HOW HOSPITALS CAN IMPROVE INFUSION TREATMENT AREAS (CONT.)

- Within reach, have a lending library of books or movies to watch.

- Cut a deal with *Netflix* or another service and provide computer notebooks where people can watch movies. Perhaps the companies who make the products would donate items for use by cancer patients.

- **When a patient finishes chemo: 1.)** Give them a card signed by the nurses. **2.)** Conduct an exit interview about foods they ate. **3.)** Ask them how their experience could have been improved — or give them a form to take home to answer these questions. **4.)** Take a picture of the patient with the nurses.

- Have an aquarium tank in the waiting room — infusion patient's morale can only be improved by seeing *living* things not images and artificial plants. Around the holidays why not have a tree, carolers or a mistletoe?

- Instead of a mortuary theme, instill the present. Have a TV playing the news. Play upbeat or contemporary music not celestial New Age crap.

- Offer popsicles or flavored cups of Italian Ice.

- **While patients are receiving chemo have a nearby lounge area where they:1.)** Gather or socialize instead of remain isolated in their chairs. **2.)** Hear lectures or see films. **3.)** Eat food. **4.)** Hold support group meetings.

- At construction sites, a lunch wagon pulls up, right? Why not a food cart offering specific meals ordered by patients and brought to their chairs or in a separate room? If you establish a special area for meals you don't have to worry about clean-ups. Get a volunteer to do it.

- Schedule chemo education programs and support groups in a nearby rooms so patients have an option to attend them *while they're receiving chemo.*

- Treat patients like they're in business class and present them with a menu so they can order from the cafeteria. Have volunteers deliver their food.

- Record seminars and give people a chance to see them on-line or make a DVD of those seminars for patients to take home or watch them during chemo.

- No volunteer musicians playing harps — stick with guitars. What about a choral group?

- In the hallways, donor nameplate pictures shouldn't haves birth and **DEATH** dates.

HOW HOSPITALS CAN IMPROVE INFUSION TREATMENT AREAS (CONT.)

- During chemo, some people lose their jobs. If their skills match the hospital's needs, how about hiring them? Or institute a job placement service to convince the hospital's high-profile corporate donors to hire survivors.

- What about organizing chemo group walks through the hospital so patients can feel like they're not lepers who have to be shielded from public view?

- Offer license plate banners. For example, Mine could say at the top "Testicular Cancer Survivor" and on the bottom: "Stanford Cancer Center."

- Brighten up the place. Have more multi-colored curtains around the patient's infusion station as well as cheerful slipcovers for recliners.

- Free parking for caregivers. Free parking for two hours to cover exams or visits. Or, give patients a token to reduce their caregiver's cost to park. Or, if an exam or waiting to get your medication takes longer than it should, cover their parking.

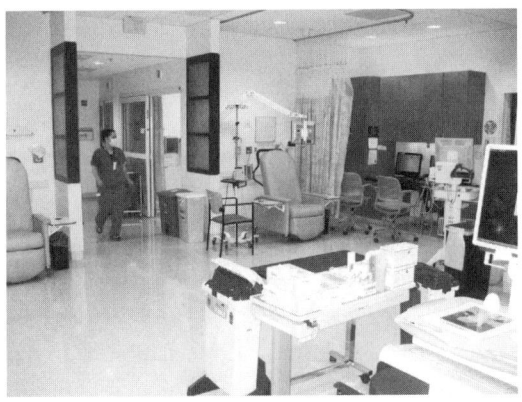

Why should chemotherapy areas look like this?
Imagine!

Brightly painted walls adorned with artwork!
Wildly patterned slipcovers over the recliners!
Colorful tiles!
Multi-colored scrubs and masks for oncology nurses!
Floor plaques with inspiring messages from donors and survivors in front of every recliner!
Hospital administrators, you don't need to consult a lawyer or form a committee.
Get your away from your desk and make this world a better place.
Leaders don't hold meetings.
Heroes just do it!

A GREAT WAY TO KNOCKOUT CANCER: THROW PUNCH LINES

CANCER IS AS REAL AS IT GETS. Funny kills serious and that's *better* then it gets. The worst people in life don't have a sense of humor and never think there's anything funny about themselves or their work, and most of the time they either run a business or are stand-up comics. Serious people incorrectly view a sense of humor as a weakness. Cancer doesn't have a sense of humor. Serious is your enemy. When seriousness overwhelms you, that's when the stress of the world, work, and bad people can bring you down. Joking was a way to keep my spirit glowing to burn away the darkness. Laughter proves cancer can't take your soul.

FRED'S CHEMO AND CANCER JOKES

- I'm worried about waking up in surgery and seeing the doctors fight over who gets the white and dark meat.

- When I first had testicular cancer I lost a testicle, so now I'm down to five.

- If you have medical insurance you get the house chemo cocktail, if not, then the oncology bartender mixes you a well drink.

- In children's hospitals they have people dress up like Spiderman, Batman, and other super heroes. That's beautiful! But what about us adults? Guys with testicular and prostate cancer, should have strippers! And women with breast cancer, male strippers!

- **Insults: A.)** Chemo attacks every rapidly reproducing cell, so your brain is safe. **B.)** Miss, Chemo is just your like your taste in men, it doesn't discriminate. **C.)** Sir, a woman dating you and getting chemo have one thing in common: having to take anti-nausea pills. **D.)** Miss, you'd get testicular cancer by having them or eating them.

- My tumor weighed four pounds — and that was just in the first trimester.

- My testosterone levels were a 6. It's supposed to be 300. This explains why I cried watching daytime talk shows about relationships and had the urge to go shopping for clothes and shoes I didn't need.

- There's a link between undescended testicles and testicular cancer. It doesn't apply to transgendered males. Their testicles aren't undescended, they're un*decided.*

- When I was getting treatment, I saw a woman who must have been pretty sexually active. They hung her chemo on a stripper's pole.

- Chemo is the only time a guy likes shrinkage.

FRED'S CHEMO AND CANCER JOKES* (CONT.)

- In a way, I hope I lost my testicles because of cancer, I hate to think I lost them because the doctors didn't like me.

- They had to remove my testicle because it was abnormal. Come on, I'm a guy. All testicles are *abnormal!*

- You know why guys hate wearing colostomy bags? We hate accessorizing. Plus it's hard to find shoes that match the color of urine or poop.

- I've never been reduced to a sexual object — well, I guess you might say after losing both testicles I'm a *reduced* sexual object. Let's say I'm marked down and come cheap.

- I've lost both testicles to cancer: **A.)** So, basically, I'm a vibrator with legs. **B.)** I should be able golf from the women's tees. **C.)** Does that mean if I wear a speedo I can show an erection and camel toe? **D.)** I'll never have to say this about testicular cancer: three times is a charm. **E.)** Now I can officially say I'm a registered Democrat. **F.)** I can check the box on any form that says "Married." **G.)** Instead of a jock, I have the option of wearing a G-string. **H.)** I have to stand between two guys to feel like I'm "hanging out." **I.)** Poker is the only way I can open with a pair — of *anything*. **J.)** So now, I'm a good-looking lesbian. **K.)** I'm just shooting air, so I can inflate a doll when I have sex with it, or gross out everyone by blowing out my birthday candles. **L.)** It might improve my disposition — I'll be less *crotch*ety. **M.)** For guys that's like getting a frontal lobotomy. **N.)** Now when I grab my crotch I don't say, "Yo!" I say, "Oh!"

- If you have too much testosterone men become argumentative, defensive and don't listen. I always thought that's what *estrogen* did to women.

- The medical term for removal of a testicle is orchiectomy. It's from the Greek "orch" which means "spay" and "hiectomy" which means "neutered."

- *(Chemo pick-up line.):* Are you in remission or are you just glad to see me?

- **I've lost both testicles, but then again, on the bright side: A.)** Never have to turn and cough again in a doctor's office. **B.)** Bring on the skinny tight jeans! **C.)** I'll never go off half-cocked. **D.)** I bet I'd do great in marathon running — less wind resistance.

- The odds of getting testicular cancer are 1 in a 100,000, and getting it the second time is slightly lower. If you get it the third time, you're an alien.

*****SPECIAL FRED TESTICLE JOKE FOR COMEDIANS:** What do you call a comedian without balls? **ANSWER:** A member of an improvisational group.

LET THE MUSIC YOU LOVE SAVE YOU

FIGHT CANCER WITH THE SOUNDTRACK OF YOUR LIFE. Go to the heart of you. The *feel* of you. The *voice* of you. Get vulnerable to the joints of what *moves* you. Arouse the spirit of play. Music is the best way to get there. These are the songs I had in heavy rotation. Their drumbeats and phrasing is where all the Freds from every year of my life dancing and stomping out cancer's hot metastasizing fire. When the singers held emotional high notes and guitars ripped hot solos and the drums pounded, driving the songs to a livelier pitch, I'd clench my fists, close my eyes and cry, trying to absorb the inspired feeling the music generated and then send is vibrating healing force throughout cells to get stronger. Sometimes when I was sitting in my recliner receiving chemo, I'd imagine myself dancing to these songs with my IV-Tower of Power in the Infusion area, spinning and wheeling around all the other Chemosabis, and then they'd join me too. And we would all go out in the hospital's hallways so everyone could see us hooked up to chemo and dancing with our IV-poles of chemo bags, showing everyone how we had nothing to hide and we were beautiful because we were *proud* of fighting for our lives!

Sing the music within you. See yourself at the age when you heard the tune. When you're alone or receiving chemo, and as weak and in as much pain and as many tears as you cry, play your music and move to it. It'll give you an edge. *Cancer can't dance, you can!* One thing I guarantee about all these songs, there's no a single harp it in any of them. If my suggestions help, great. But find yours.

FRED'S CHEMO PLAY LIST: UPBEAT TUNES THAT GOT ME GOING

- Right Back Where We Started From – Maxine Nightingale
- Wishin' and Hopin' – Dusty Springfield
- Mickey – Toni Basil
- What a Feeling – Irene Cara
- Denise – Randy and The Rainbows
- Shake Rattle and Roll – Joe Turner
- This Whole World & *The Surfer Girl* album – The Beach Boys
- You Can't Hurry Love – Supremes
- Castanets – Alejandro Escovedo
- That's Life – Frank Sinatra
- Holiday Road – Lindsay Buckingham
- I'm All Right – Kenny Loggins
- 500 Miles – The Proclaimers Runaway Train – Soul Asylum
- Bittersweet – Big Head Todd
- Get Rhythm & Riding In My Car & Beverly – NRBQ
- My Love – Petula Clark
- Concrete and Clay – Unit 4+2

FRED'S CHEMO PLAY LIST: UPBEAT TUNES THAT GOT ME GOING (CONT.)

- My Pledge of Love – Joe Jeffrey Group
- It Came Out Of The Sky – Credence Clearwater Revival
- Passionate Kisses & Ten Year Ache – Rosanne Cash
- Psychotic Reaction – Count Five
- Island In The Sun – Weezer
- Any Way You Want – Harvey Faqua
- I Love This Bar – Toby Keith
- Let's Twist & Do The Hucklebuck – Chubby Checker
- Help Yourself – Tom Jones
- Better Things – The Kinks
- Tonight The Streets Are Ours – Richard Hawley
- Working My Way Back To You – The Four Seasons
- I Can't Stop Hurting Myself – Greg Kihn
- Lightning Strikes & I'm Gonna Make You Mine – Lou Christie
- If I Had A Hammer – Trini Lopez
- That Thing You Do! – The Wonders
- Don't Go Back To Rockville – R.E.M
- Mountain of Love – Johnny Rivers
- Tenderness – General Public
- Man In The Mirror – Michael Jackson
- Photograph – Ringo
- I Would – Fred Eaglesmith
- Sign, Sealed, Delivered & I Ain't Going To Stand For It – Stevie Wonder
- Honestly Sincere – *Bye Bye Birdie* soundtrack
- Beautiful Day – U2
- Go All The Way – The Raspberries
- You've Lost That Lovin' Feeling – Righteous Brothers
- I Will Dare – The Replacements
- Devil With A Blue Dress On – Mitch Ryder and The Detroit Wheels
- Build Me Up Buttercup – Foundations
- Dinner With Drac – John Zacherle
- From Small Things (Big Things One Day Come), Rosalita, Fourth of July Asbury Park (Sandy), Ain't Good Enough For you, Out In The Street & Promised Land, Badlands – Bruce Springsteen
- Higher and Higher – Jackie Wilson
- Oh How Happy – Shades of Blue
- Help Yourself – Tom Jones
- Let's Stay Together – Al Green
- Everybody Loves Somebody Sometime – Dean Martin
- Reach Out For Me – Dionne Warwick
- 1-2-3 Red Light – 1910 Fruit Gum Company

FRED'S CHEMO PLAY LIST: UPBEAT TUNES THAT GOT ME GOING (CONT.)

- It Ain't What You Eat It's The Way You Chew It & Flying Saucer Rock 'n' Roll & Everyday – Sleepy LaBeef
- Donna The Prima Donna – Dion and The Belmonts
- Hey Hey Hey – Michael Franti & Spearhead
- What I Did For Love – Chorus Line Soundtrack
- The Dead Heart – Midnight Oil
- Power of Love – Huey Lewis and The News
- Spirit In The Sky – Norman Greenbaum
- Dance With Me Tonight – Hugh Grant
- Let's Work Together – Canned Heat
- God's Radar – Dixie Hummingbirds
- Change The World – Eric Clapton
- Magic Moments – Perry Como
- There She Goes – The La's
- I'm Mr. Blue & Come Softly To Me – Fleetwoods
- The Mouse – Soupy Sales
- Groovy Kind of Love – Mindbenders
- Human Wheels – John Mellencamp
- Half A Boy And Half A Man – Nick Lowe
- The Image of a Girl – The Safaris
- Expressway To Your Heart – The Soul Survivors
- Sweet Soul Music – Arthur Conley
- I Got Rhythm – Happenings
- Cara Mia – Jay and The Americans
- Hold On! I'm Coming! & Soul Man – Sam & Dave
- Blessed – Elton John
- MacArthur Park – Richard Harris
- Hold me, Thrill Me, Kiss Me – Mel Carter
- Is It So Strange & All Shook Up – Elvis Presley
- I Fought The Law – Bobby Fuller
- Cry Me A River – Joe Cocker
- Double Shot of My Baby's Love – Swinging Medallions
- She's My Baby – Traveling Wilburys
- I'm Yours – Jason Mraz
- Cool Jerk – Capitols
- I can See The Pines Are Dancing – A.A. Bondy
- **Honorable Mention:** James Brown on the T.A.M.I Show DVD.

Want *more*
Fred in your head?
(Turn the page.)

Blind Guys Break 80...

"What a story! I really, really liked it. Took *Blind Guys Break 80* on a plane flight from California to England. It was the fastest flight ever. That's my quote!"

– **Huey Lewis,** *rock singer, 10-handicap golfer*

"Fred Reiss did for golf what he previously did for surfing — given us a hip, insider's story told with a wicked sense of humor."

– **Chris Miller,** *National Lampoon author of Animal House*

"Fred Reiss has done something pretty cool with *Blind Guys Break 80*. He's turned a golf course into not just a metaphor for life but an entertaining stage where characters crack wicked jokes and utter deep truths. Imagine teeing it up in a foursome of John Daly, Martha Stewart, David Mamet and George Carlin. Then imagine a 19th hole therapy session with them. That sort of explains what Reiss is up to here — but that doesn't begin to touch on the sweet family drama at the heart of it all. I give this book four strokes a side and four stars out of four."

– **Mark Purdy,** *sports columnist, San Jose Mercury News*

Surf.Com pen-award-winning novel...

"With *Gidget Must Die* and now *Surf.Com*, Fred Reiss has emerged as a sort of surfy Hunter S. Thompson, a vicious, merciless, ridiculous social documentarian with a distinct flair for drawing unforgettable characters. Fred Reiss is nuts. But mainly, he is very, very funny."

– **Alan Weisbecker,** *author of Searching for Captain Zero*

Gidget Must Die...

"Gidget Must Die is a witty, surreal, and insulting text laced with keen perceptions and dead-on portraits of our sport's archetypes. Make no mistake about it, this guy Fred Reiss is sick. I recommend GMD for a hundred or so other reasons."

– **Drew Kampion,** *editor of Surfer's Path*

"Fred made me laugh and squirm through the Malibu culturati. I choked on the asphalt fumes of PCH, and breathed the salt spray of the "Bu" again. I'm with him in the pre-dawn perfection, taking off until — but let Reiss tell it. He'll suck you over the falls with his wild surf yarn (Or is it?)."

– **John Severson,** *founder of Surfer Magazine*

Insult And Live!...

"If you've ever been late with a comeback, BUY Reiss."

– **Playboy Magazine**

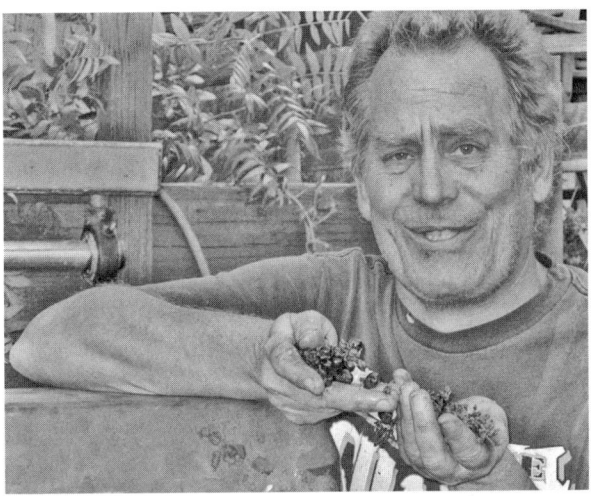

FRED HAS HARVESTED WINE (*above:* He survived cancer to enjoy the great 2012 Santa Cruz Mountain harvest.). He was treated, tagged and released by the great folks at the Stanford Cancer Center in Palo Alto, CA. Fred worked as a talk-radio host and stand-up comic. Back in the day, Fred spent several years as a reporter at the *Fairfield Citizen-News* and the *Danbury News-Times* in Connecticut until he had testicular cancer (One testicle plucked, he's was down to five.). After being given a second chance to live, Fred quit journalism, lit out for California to surf, do stand-up comedy, make wine and write. Fred has performed in Bakersfield, Yuba City and on national TV (See "Love me" *YouTube*.). He won a PEN award for his novel *Surf.Com*. Fred fills in the gaps hoping to get stronger to surf again, doing volunteer speaking work for the American Cancer Society and Relay For Life. He gets vertical working the tasting rooms at the Beauregard Vineyards and MJA Vineyards, or helping out at the Hallcrest Winery in the Santa Cruz Mountains. He's held enriching dead-end jobs in advertising, a bank, a Florida mental facility, a bed & breakfast, a warehouse, a surf shop, several radio stations. He's even been a camp counselor, painter, cleaned toilets, shrink-wrapped pallets in a warehouse, bar-backed, harvested and made wine, substitute taught and instructed tennis. At age 57, Fred got testicular cancer again (Now he's down to *four*.). After being given a third chance to live, Fred wrote this book to help others reduce their suffering, improve their care and overcome The Big C. He lives with Laurie, three rescued cool cats named Bogie, Groucho and Brooksie, as well as a high-maintenance barking poop-machine rescued dog named Seven.

Fred blogs at http://fredforyourhead.wordpress.com. You can purchase his books at www.fredforyourhead.com. Check out his *YouTube* vids.

Thank you for your support. Best of health to all you know. Live forever as long as you can.

Get More Fred In Your Head

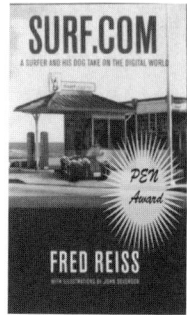

PEN-Award Winning Novel

Surf.Com

The dot-commers are ruining Santa Cruz. The only force left to defeat them is a surfer, a dog, and a van. But when the surfer falls in love with a dot-com girl, things get gnarly. **Also an eBook at Amazon.com.**
$16.95

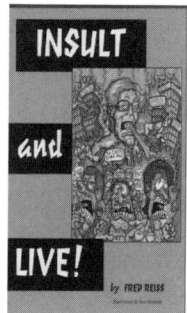

The Book of Slams …

Insult and Live!

1,000 stage-tested insults. Fred was an insult comic. Appeared on national TV. In this twisted magnum of an opus, he identifies every loser in the world. Hot flamers to slam jerks so you can man-up and truly live.
$16.95

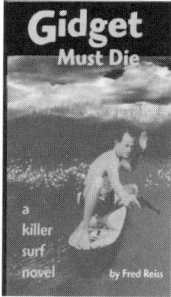

Killer Surf Novel with a Heart

Gidget Must Die

It's thirty years later, a surf legend from the fifties returns to Malibu to kill everyone in the Gidget movie for ruining his beloved surf spot. **Also an eBook at Amazon.com.**
$14.95

Get More Fred In Your Head

Surf Sci-Fi Novel by an Author in Remission.

ALIENS! SURF! SANTA CRUZ!

A surfer learns aliens are trying extract Santa Cruz's stoke to transport it their planet. He's not giving up his stoke and his surf spots to a bunch of kook trannie aliens.
Available as an eBook at Amazon.com.
$15.95

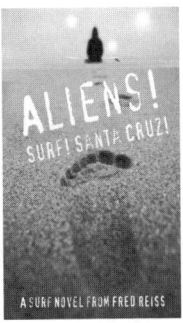

The ebook of Slams...

INSULTS TO GO

Wow! 2,000-plus insults. Over 1,000 flamers from Fred's act and never put into book form until now. Includes illustrations and slams from the previous book. These.
Only available as an eBook at Amazon.com.
$9.95

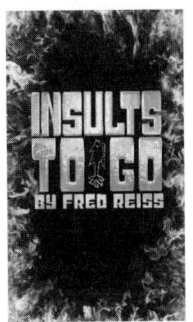

Long Day's Journey on the Back Nine.

BLIND GUYS BREAK 80

Cloudy is a middle-aged loser who wants to earn his father's respect by improving at golf. As he struggles to find his true swing. Cloudy discovers his blindness in golf and life can only be overcome with his mother's love, the guiding spirit of Freehold, NJ, and Herb Alpert & the Tijuana Brass.
Available as an ebook at Amazon.com.
$15.95

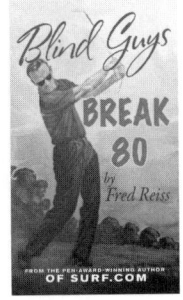

Order books at fredforyourhead.com.

Head for Fred: Get a signed book with an inscription from the author. Send a check for price of the book, plus $3.95 for shipping and handling to Fred Reiss, PO Box 733, Mount Hermon, CA, 95041.
Thank you for your support.

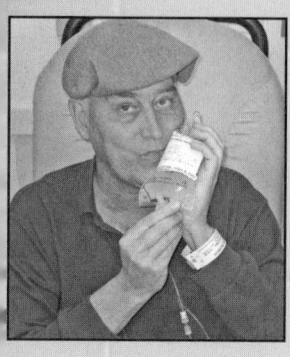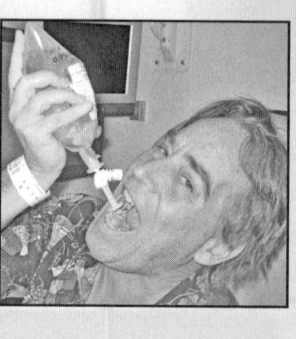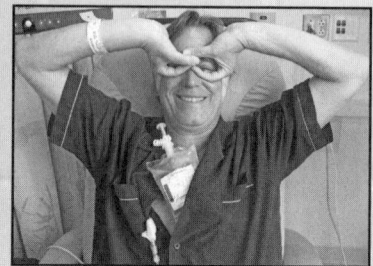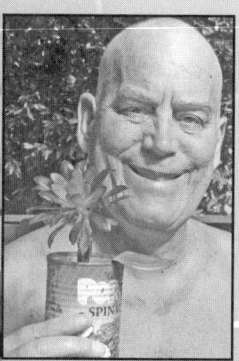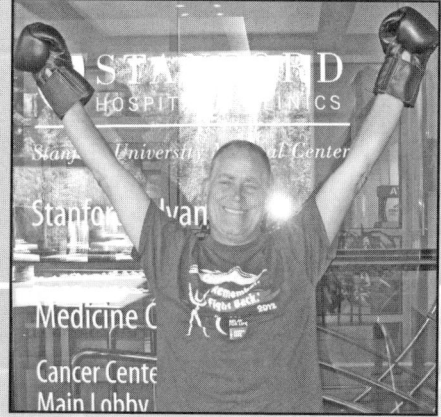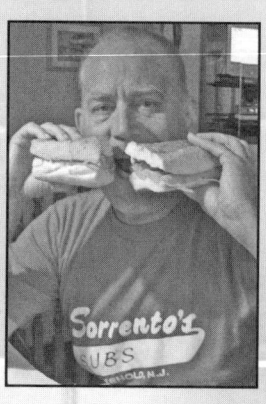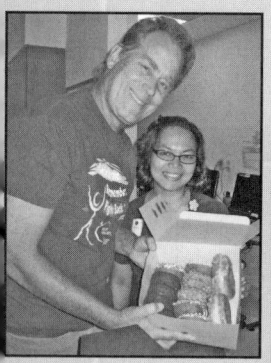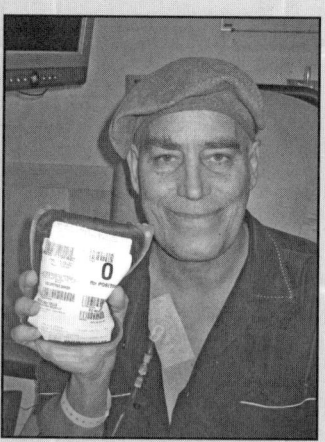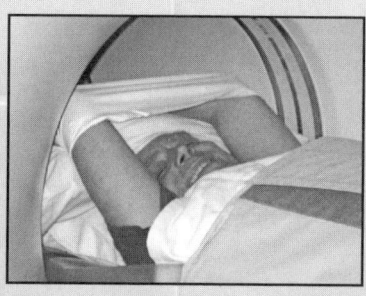